Respiratory Medicine

Series Editors

Sharon I. S. Rounds
Brown University
Providence, RI, USA

Anne Dixon
University of Vermont, Larner College of Medicine
Burlington, VT, USA

Lynn M. Schnapp
University of Wisconsin - Madison
Madison, WI, USA

More information about this series at http://www.springer.com/series/7665

Cynthia D. Brown • Erin Crowley
Editors

Transitioning Care from Pediatric to Adult Pulmonology

Ensuring Best Practices and Optimal Outcomes

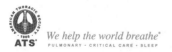

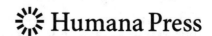

Editors
Cynthia D. Brown
Division of Pulmonary, Critical Care,
Occupational, and Sleep Medicine
Indiana University School of Medicine
Indianapolis, IN
USA

Erin Crowley
Department of Pulmonary, Critical Care,
and Sleep Medicine
Wyoming Medical Center
Casper, WY
USA

ISSN 2197-7372   ISSN 2197-7380   (electronic)
Respiratory Medicine
ISBN 978-3-030-68690-1   ISBN 978-3-030-68688-8   (eBook)
https://doi.org/10.1007/978-3-030-68688-8

This Humana imprint is published by the registered company Springer Nature Switzerland AG
The registered company address is: Gewerbestrasse 11, 6330 Cham, Switzerland

Contents

Contributors

Jordan D. Awerbach, MD, PhD Phoenix Children's Hospital, Department of Cardiology, Phoenix, AZ, USA

Sarah E. Bauer, MD Riley Hospital for Children, Division of Pediatric Pulmonology, Allergy and Sleep Medicine, Indianapolis, IN, USA

Cecily L. Betz, PhD, RN, FAAN Keck School of Medicine, Department of Pediatrics, University of Southern California, Los Angeles, CA, USA

Cynthia D. Brown, MD Division of Pulmonary, Critical Care, Occupational, and Sleep Medicine, Indiana University School of Medicine, Indianapolis, IN, USA

Jeanette P. Brown, MD, PhD Internal Medicine Division of Pulmonary, Critical Care & Occupational Pulmonary, University of Utah, Salt Lake City, UT, USA

Jennifer L. Butcher, PhD Michigan Medicine C.S. Mott Children's Hospital, Ann Arbor, MI, USA

Pi Chun Cheng, MD Division of Pulmonary Medicine, Children's Hospital of Philadelphia, Philadelphia, PA, USA

Katherine Alex Despotes, MD The University of North Carolina at Chapel Hill, Chapel Hill, NC, USA

Wayne J. Franklin, MD Phoenix Children's Hospital, Department of Cardiology, Phoenix, AZ, USA

Jennifer L. Goralski, MD The University of North Carolina at Chapel Hill, Chapel Hill, NC, USA

Kathleen S. Irby, MD Internal Medicine-Pediatrics, University of Utah, Salt Lake City, UT, USA

Stephen Kirkby, MD Division of Pulmonary, Critical Care & Sleep Medicine, Department of Internal Medicine, The Ohio State University Wexner Medical Center, Columbus, OH, USA

Section of Pulmonary Medicine, Nationwide Children's Hospital, Columbus, OH, USA

Nadia L. Krupp, MD Riley Hospital for Children, Division of Pediatric Pulmonology, Allergy and Sleep Medicine, Indianapolis, IN, USA

Karen Lowton, PhD Department of Sociology, University of Sussex, Brighton, UK

Cory Powers, MD Departments of Internal Medicine and Pediatrics, Indiana University School of Medicine, Indianapolis, IN, USA

Rachel Quaney, MD Division of Pulmonary, Critical Care & Sleep Medicine, Department of Internal Medicine, The Ohio State University Wexner Medical Center, Columbus, OH, USA

Michael M. Rey, MD, MSHP Division of Pulmonary, Allergy, & Critical Care Medicine, University of Pennsylvania and University of Pennsylvania Perelman School of Medicine, Philadelphia, PA, USA

Division of Pulmonary and Critical Care Medicine, Corporal Michael J. Crescenz VA Medical Center, Philadelphia, PA, USA

Lisa A. Schwartz, PhD Division of Oncology, Children's Hospital of Philadelphia and University of Pennsylvania Perelman School of Medicine, Philadelphia, PA, USA

Dava Szalda, MD, MSHP Division of Oncology, Children's Hospital of Philadelphia and University of Pennsylvania Perelman School of Medicine, Philadelphia, PA, USA

Part I
General Principles of Transition Care

Chapter 1
Development of Healthcare Transition Policy and Concepts

Cecily L. Betz

Introduction

The evolution of the field of healthcare transition (HCT) emanated in part from the increasing numbers of adolescents with childhood-acquired disabilities and chronic conditions who entered into adulthood. Ninety percent of children born with chronic conditions are now projected to survive into adulthood [58]. According to recent estimates, approximately one million adolescents with chronic conditions reach adulthood and enter the adult system of health care [47]. Of the number of adolescents entering the adult healthcare system, approximately 3% are identified as having complex medical needs, referred to in pediatric care as children with medical complexity (CMC). This subgroup of adolescents with complex medical needs are so described as they have significant functional limitations (i.e., technology dependent; non-ambulatory); have extensive needs for a myriad of specialty medical services; and have disproportionate health utilization compared to typical usage of health care services as they are at higher risk for hospitalization and emergency department visits [1, 17, 35, 36].

The evident, yet unexpected, surge of this new population of adolescents and young adults with complex healthcare needs has created new challenges for both pediatric and adult healthcare systems. These ever growing and pressing developments have been exacerbated by the inadequacy of service models for facilitating the exit from pediatric care and the access to adult care as no formal transfer linkages between them has existed. Problematic as well has been the lack of preparation programs to support adolescents and young adults and their families for the transition from pediatric to adult health care. Findings of the 2016 National Survey of

C. L. Betz (✉)
Keck School of Medicine, Department of Pediatrics, University of Southern California, Los Angeles, CA, USA
e-mail: cbetz@chla.usc.edu

© Springer Nature Switzerland AG 2021
C. D. Brown, E. Crowley (eds.), *Transitioning Care from Pediatric to Adult Pulmonology*, Respiratory Medicine,
https://doi.org/10.1007/978-3-030-68688-8_1

Children's Health (NSCH) revealed the vast majority of adolescents with (83%) and without (86%) special healthcare needs (SHCN) had not received HCT preparation according to national performance metrics [38]. Furthermore, providers in both sectors of this system of health care have been ill equipped to provide the services needed for preparing this new population of medically complex patients to leave pediatric care and to access the care of healthcare professionals positioned to receive them [53].

The intent of this chapter is to provide the reader with a historical perspective about the early roots and beginnings of the field of HCT practice and research. To accomplish this purpose, the narrative will begin with the causative factors that created the needs for this new model of service for young adults and adults with childhood-acquired long-term conditions. These factors created the recognition of the need for change as well as the challenges in effecting the development and implementation of HCT service models. In essence, a massive reshaping of the exit portal of the pediatric system of care together with a conduit of entrance into adult care was needed as historical policy-related precedents were formidable opposing factors to effect change. The professional and governmental developments that ensued during the seminal stages of the field will be presented, ending with a "snapshot" of current developments in research and practice and the implications for the future.

Survival Rates of Children with Long-Term Conditions: Then and Now

The advances in the science and care of children born with congenital disorders and those diagnosed with long-term conditions within the last generation alone have brought remarkable changes in the treatment and long-term management of this vulnerable pediatric population. The dramatic contrasts in survivability as described here are illustrative. In the late 1930s, more than 70% of children diagnosed with cystic fibrosis (CF) died before the age of 2 years. Today, life expectancy for individuals born with CF extends into the mid and late 40s [18, 19, 21, 66]. In 1970, less than 50% of adolescents diagnosed with sickle cell disease survived into adulthood [64]. Recent reports indicate that 93.9% of with sickle cell anemia (HbSS) or sickle 0-thalassemia (HbSβ°) survive into adulthood with a medium age of survival over 50. Nearly all (98.4%) of those with sickle hemoglobin C disease (HbSC) or sickle thalassemia (HbSβ⁺) have survival rates comparable to the typical population [14, 15, 59].

Prior to the neurosurgical treatment of infants born with spina bifida (SB), most often it was considered as a fatal diagnosis [37]. The survival rates of infants born with SB in the 1960s and 1970s improved with more aggressive treatment approaches enabling more favorable prognosis beyond infancy and childhood [28, 41, 46, 54]. Adulthood survival rate estimates, although dependent on the level of SB involvement, are now reported as 60% for survival into the 20s [60]. More recent studies have reported survival rates of 39% for age 40 and 32% for age 50 that are based on longitudinal study of cohort of children born (between 1963 and 1971) in the United Kingdom [54, 55].

In the 1960s, for children diagnosed with Duchenne muscular dystrophy (DMD), life expectancy was estimated to extend to adolescence [23]. Survival rates have been reported up to midlife [32].

The advances in treatments and long-term management of children diagnosed with long-term conditions have enabled their survival into adulthood as illustrated in this discussion. The improvements described of the selected long-term conditions profiled here are indicative of hopeful yet realistic expectations for the future for children with long-term conditions.

Age Parameters and Pediatric Policies of Care

As described in this section, the age parameters defining the pediatric scope of practice for children and adolescents has undergone major revisions since the organizational inception of pediatrics. The formalization of the defining boundaries of pediatric care has been an influencing factor for understanding long-standing perspectives toward aging adolescents and young adults.

Beginning in 1938 and subsequently, pediatrics has delimited the age parameters for clinical practice. The earliest age parameters were identified in 1938, and "the practice of pediatrics begins at birth and extends well into adolescence and in most cases it will terminate between the sixteenth and eighteenth year of life (AAP [2, p. 266] as cited in AAP [3, p. 463]). In 1972, the age range of pediatric care was expanded with this statement: "The responsibility of pediatrics may therefore begin during pregnancy and usually terminates by 21 years of age" (AAP, Council on Child Health [40, p. 463]). The age limit of 21 was reaffirmed in 1988 with the proviso that care could be extended beyond age 21 for those with a chronic illness or disability "…if mutually agreeable to the pediatrician, the patient, and when appropriate the patient's family…" (AAP, Council on Child and Adolescent Health, [4, p. 738]).

The most recent AAP statement, Age Limits of Pediatrics, published in 2017 departs from previous policy enumerations of age limitations. This policy document suggests that the upper age limit of 21 "…is an arbitrary demarcation line for adolescence" [26, p. 2]. Instead, this newest policy iteration advocates that specialty care pediatricians consider the condition-related needs of patients rather than the usual terminal age of care at 21 years in circumstances wherein capacity of adult specialty care is limited. Under these circumstances, a hybrid model involving collaboration with primary care providers is encouraged.

This policy change in age parameters is predicated on the revised understanding of adolescent brain development, contemporary societal trends of adolescent and emerging adult development, and the complex care needs of those with SHCN and disabilities [8, 22]. The issue of the clinical capacity of adult providers has been raised repeatedly in the pediatric literature as it pertains to providing specialized care and understanding of the psychosocial dynamics of living with a childhood-acquired disability/chronic condition [53]. Surveys of specialty adult providers' willingness and preparedness to receive adults with childhood-acquired disabilities/chronic conditions acknowledge the challenges but have referred to issues on the pediatric side that are seen as barriers to promoting the smooth uninterrupted transfer and establishment of care with adult providers. These challenges include insufficient/nonexistent communication initiated by pediatric providers with the adult counterparts and patients who are ill prepared and not health literate to manage and assume responsibilities for their own healthcare needs [16, 57].

Healthcare Transition Policy Initiatives

In its infancy as a practice field and area of study, important initiatives were promulgated that spurred the development of HCT. The professional associations as the American Academy of Pediatrics and the Society of Adolescent Medicine were leaders in calling the attention of not only pediatricians but their colleagues in adult medicine and their interdisciplinary pediatric colleagues of this service need for adolescents and young adults with and without SHCN to effect improved outcomes for these populations. Investments by the federal government were pivotal to spurring the early and ongoing developments in HCT.

Leadership Efforts of Surgeon General C. Everett Koop

Against the backdrop of this significant public health issue, under the leadership of the US Surgeon General, C. Everett Koop, and in collaboration with major pediatric and adolescent health organizations, advocacy groups, and federal partners, HCT for adolescents with chronic conditions was acknowledged as a pressing national service need nearly 40 years ago [13, 34, 45]. Two national invitational conferences were held to address the issue and formulate a national action agenda. The first 1984 HCT conference, *Youth with Disability: The Transition Years*, and, later, the 1989 Surgeon General's conference, *Growing Up and Getting Medical Care: Youth with Special Health Care Needs* brought together the clinical experts from pediatrics, nursing, and psychology; policy analysts; representatives of medical associations and organizations; and state, federal, and private sector administrators to address the national public health issue [13, 34, 45].

The 1989 Surgeon General's meeting explored the scope of the problem as presented by invited experts that included the barriers associated with transition to and the establishment of access to the adult system of care, its financing, and the capacity limitations of interdisciplinary pediatric and adult healthcare professionals to engage in transition services [34, 45]. Several examples of piloted transition programs in the United States were presented as well as the exemplary model of comprehensive services and supports for individuals in the Netherlands that included healthcare, employment training and placements, housing, and community living. The action plan generated by this conference included:

- Development of care guidelines for transition services
- Exploration of options for reimbursement for transition services
- Development of transition service models based on a family-centered care framework
- Provision of education and training on transition for interdisciplinary healthcare professionals to enhance capacity and competence
- Research to develop and implement evidence-based transition models

HCT Initiatives of Pediatric and Adolescent Organizations

Several years later in 1993, a position paper on transition was produced by the Society of Adolescent Medicine, entitled *Transition from Child-Centered to Adult Health-Care Systems for Adolescents with Chronic Conditions* [13]. This landmark publication, one of the most highly cited publications on the topic, contained an overview of the research and practice in this emerging field of HCT. As acknowledged in this article, there were few service models implemented and tested, limited in part by the paucity of research conducted at the time. For example, the authors noted "Adequate measures exist; however, they have not been used in any study of transitional programs" (Blum et al., p. 570). Of note, the definition of transition offered in this publication has become predominant as a conceptual explanation, "...as the purposeful, planned movement of adolescents and young adults with chronic physical and medical conditions from child-centered to adult-oriented health-care systems" [13, p. 570]. This early definition of HCT focused on the transfer procedure associated with HCT process.

Later, in September 1994, an invitational conference on transition entitled *Moving On: Transition from Pediatric to Adult Health Care* was hosted [12]. The purpose of this conference was to convene an international group of experts in adolescent and adult care who had experience with transition. Commissioned papers from this conference appeared in the *Journal of Adolescent Health* that addressed pertinent issues on HCT. Of interest, one of the earliest clinical commentaries, entitled *Between Two Worlds: Bridging the Cultures of Child Health and Adult Medicine*, authored by an internist appeared in this issue [61]. This was one of the first articles published by a non-pediatric professional pertaining to HCT. The cultural contrasts between these divergent service models were explicated in terms of the challenges associated with the transfer of care. Conference recommendations focused on implications for service, training, quality improvement, and research. Importantly, transition was conceptualized not as an event, but rather as a long-term process beginning at diagnosis based upon a family-centered framework of care. Interestingly, the four models of care highlighted for recommendations were based on joint service models involving pediatric and adult providers that focused on the transfer process: (a) disease specific; (b) generic; (c) primary care; and (d) single site (Box 1.1).

Box 1.1 Early Proposed Models of Care

Disease specific	Transfer of care is initiated in the pediatric specialty program followed by joint team/clinic of pediatric and adult specialty providers before transfer to the adult specialty service.
Generic	Transfer of care is coordinated by the primary care pediatrician in consultation with specialty providers followed by the transfer to adolescent primary care team in consultation with specialty providers followed by transfer to internist who coordinates care with referrals to specialty providers.
Primary care	Care is coordinated by general practitioner in consultation with pediatric and adult specialty care providers as consultants.
Single site model	The continuum of care is provided in one setting: seamless healthcare organization.

Summary of Recommendations [67]

In 1996, the American Academy of Pediatrics issued its first policy statement on HCT, jointly authored by the Committee on Children with Disabilities and the Committee on Adolescence [6]. Unlike the Society of Adolescent Medicine's position paper published in 1993, this document did not define HCT. Rather, issues pertaining to achieving developmental milestones associated with adulthood and the pediatrician's role in facilitating their achievements were presented. Practice responsibilities of pediatricians for transition planning and support were enumerated such as strategies to use in promoting the adolescent's independence pertaining to self-care, community living, and fiscal matters. Postsecondary goals associated with education and employment were identified as relevant pediatric practice concerns in providing guidance and resource information to adolescents and their families. Pragmatic discussions pertaining to insurance coverage once eligibility for pediatric coverage terminates and enrollment/redetermination in various Social Security Administration programs such as Supplemental Security Income (SSI) and Social Security Disability Insurance (SSDI) were covered.

Ambiguity is evident in this early policy statement as it pertains to hospitalization during this period of transition from pediatric to adult care, as several recommendations were offered to address the needs of the new population of patients for providers who had limited clinical experience in the provision of their care [6]. An evident recommendation is made for training of adult staff involved with inpatient care of adolescent/young adult patients with SHCN involving condition management. A period of joint management by the pediatrician and adult provider is suggested during the period of transition to care provided solely by adult healthcare providers. Another yet uncommon recommendation is suggested that primary care pediatricians "..seek admitting privileges to the adult unit to ensure their continuing participation as the primary attending physician or as a consultant" [6, p. 1205]. Of importance during this period of transition is the adolescent's/young adult's full participation and involvement in transition planning that is based on their preferences and needs.

HCT Consensus Statement

A turning point was achieved in policymaking in the HCT field with the publication of the first consensus policy document, entitled *A Consensus Statement on Health Care Transitions for Young Adults with Special Health Care Needs* issued by the AAP, American Academy of Family Physicians (AAFP), and American College of Physicians (ACP)-American Society of Internal Medicine (ASIM) [5]. Although the agreed-upon recommendations were circumscribed, the ramifications were significant. The *Consensus Statement* provided a collective acknowledgement of necessity to facilitating the transfer of care for young adults with SHCN from pediatric to adult care. Furthermore, there was collaborative agreement that this process required informed and skilled professionals involved in the process on both sides – the sending and receiving ends of the process. The importance of this *Consensus Statement* was the collective involvement of major pediatric and adult professional associations to craft an agreement and acknowledgement of this field of practice and the necessity of moving forward to craft new models of collaboration to effect improved outcomes for adolescents and young adults with SHCN.

2011 Clinical Report Issued by AAP, AAFP, and ACP

Nearly a decade later, this professional coalition composed of the AAP, AAFP, and ACP published clinical practice guidance, the *Clinical Report*, for implementing HCT services for youth and young adults [7]. Of clinical relevance, although the preceding *Consensus Statement* was directed specifically to address the clinical challenges of youth and young adults with SHCN's HCT from pediatric to adult health care, this *Clinical Report* was broader in scope. This clinical algorithm was designed for application for *all* youth and young adults including those with SHCN. This algorithm of the clinical guideline, based upon a patient and family-centered model of primary care, included three dimensions of practice-preventive care, acute illness care, and chronic condition management (CCM). Developers of the algorithm noted that this guide could be applied to specialty practice as well. This *Clinical Report* was designed not only as an algorithm for the provision of HCT services, but importantly serves as the template from which subsequent AAP publications are developed pertaining to this field of practice, research, and quality improvement.

Noteworthy elements of the *Clinical Report* begin with the distinction between transition and transfer of care. The transition process as enumerated in this document is a lengthy process of clinical monitoring, service coordination and referral, and youth and young adult education to foster health literacy and CCM. Unlike the previous *Consensus Statement* wherein the age range focused on the transfer of care period, the *Clinical Report* recommended the age of 12 for initiating HCT, although an earlier age for youth with SHCN is cited as appropriate [7].

For the first time, the algorithm of the *Clinical Report* provided concise guidance as to the action steps to be undertaken along the developmental continuum to foster and support the youth's and young adult's transition and transfer of care. Previously, guidance published by pediatric and adolescent medicine professional associations broadly stated areas of practice emphasis pertaining to this new and developing field of care for the ever increasing youth and young adult population with SHCN. This *Clinical Report* also directed attention to the roles and responsibilities of the adult medical home providers who receive youth and young adults. Paramount considerations of the transfer procedure are the identification of adult providers who are prepared to receive the generational group of adolescents and young adults and the transmission of medical information to new service providers so as to proceed smoothly and competently with care.

2018 Clinical Report *Issued by AAP, AAFP, and ACP*

More recently, an update of the 2011 *Clinical Report* was published in 2018 [69]. This *Clinical Report* revision reflects more current developments in the field with the proliferation of literature now being generated as evident with the research being produced using more rigorous designs and methodologies (refer to State of Research, Clinical Practice, and Beyond for additional information).

The 2018 *Clinical Report* provides new attention to the *Six Core Elements for Pediatric and Adult Care* (described in greater detail below), enlarged scope of HCT practice, special populations, reimbursement options, and training resources for pediatric and adult providers who provide services to youth and young adults with SHCN. These recommendations reflect the progress and development in the HCT field.

Federal Initiative: Title V Programs for Children with Special Health Care Needs

In this section, several federal initiatives will be presented that have influenced the need for and served to foster the development and implementation of HCT resources and service models in the United States. This review will begin with the establishment of the Crippled Children's Service, a federal program in 1935, described in detail below and conclude with current resources available for youth and young adults, families, and healthcare and non-healthcare professionals.

Title V Programs for Children with Special Health Care Needs

There are many federal programs whose mission is to address the needs of children, adolescents, and young adults with SHCN. Foremost, among these programs is the Title V Program, a block grant program of the Maternal Child Health Program of the US Department of Health and Human Services. Historically, the Title V Program was first established in 1935 through the authorization of the Social Security Act in Title V of the legislation that allocated block grant funding to states for health and welfare services for women and children that included maternity and infant care. A portion of Title V funding was allocated for children with chronic conditions, then known as the Crippled Children's Service (CCS) [9, 30]. The vast majority of children initially served through CCS had orthopedic impairments; subsequently other diagnostic groups of children were served that included those with congenital heart disorders and rheumatic fever [31].

Fifty years later in 1985, with the passage of Public Law (PL) 99-272, the name of Crippled Children's Service was changed to the Program for Children with Special Health Care Needs (CSHCN). Later, amendments to the Title V were effected in the Omnibus Budget Reconciliation Act (OBRA) (PL 101-239) in 1989 which expanded the mission of the program. These programmatic changes required states to allocate 30% of the block grant funds for children with SHCN. Concomitant with this requirement was the directive to create a system of care that would better serve this population of children, youth, and their families. This new provision stipulated that the service system was to provide care that was family-centered, community-based, and coordinated [29, 30].

In an effort to create greater accountability of the grant funding provided, new reporting requirements were enacted in the (OBRA) of 1989 [33]. These new programmatic guidelines specified that a system of performance standards incorporating measurable metrics (i.e., annual goals) to monitor progress with Title V Maternal and Child Health Services Block Grant funding be established at the federal level by the Maternal and Child Health Bureau (MCHB). Initially, 18 National Performance Measures (NPM) (later reduced to 15) were developed that were based upon the legislative requirements of the Title V Programs. The 1997 programmatic areas covered maternal child health, adolescent services, and CSHCN. Each of the 50 states, the District of Columbia, and the 9 territories selected 8 NPM from the list of 18 NPM. Concurrently with the development of NPM for all of the Title V Programs, the Maternal and Child Health Bureau (MCHB) formulated six core outcomes for CSHCN. These initial core outcomes were integrated in the NPM for CSHCN listed in Box 1.2.

Box 1.2 Core Outcomes for CSHCN

No.	Core Outcomes
1.	Families of SCHCN will partner in decision-making and will be satisfied with the services that they receive.
2.	CSHCN will receive coordinated, ongoing, comprehensive care within a medical home.
3.	Families of CSHCN will have adequate private and/or public insurance to pay for the services that they need.
4.	Children will be screened early and continuously for special healthcare needs.
5.	Community-based service systems will be organized so that families can use them easily.
6.	Youth with special healthcare needs will receive the services necessary to make transitions to adult life, including adult health care, work, and independence.

McPherson et al. [48, p. 1539]

National Performance Measure # 12: Transition

In 2015, the national performance measurement system was substantially revised. Transition continues as one of the NPM as it was "…considered crucial to the development of a well-functioning system of care for children with special health care needs" [33, p. 950]. However, the revised transition NPM is more inclusive in scope in terms of addressing the entire adolescent population but more narrowly focused on health care in contrast to earlier NPM, which was broader as work and independence were addressed: NPM # 12: *Transition (percent of adolescents with and without special healthcare needs who received services necessary to make transitions to adult health care)*. The rational for delimiting the scope of this NPM was the extent to which it could be measured with an accessible and reliable data source.

Currently, there are 36 states and territories that have selected NPM # 12: Transition as a NPM as presented below in Box 1.3.

Healthy People: **National Health Report Cards and CSHCN**

Healthy People (HP) reports of 2000, 2010, and 2020 provide the template for guiding and assessing the nation's progress in achieving health goals and objectives of pertinence to the US public [56]. Hence, the HP reports are broad and comprehensive in scope as health issues of concern for the American public across the lifespan are addressed. Beginning in *HP 2000*, objectives for CSHCN were integrated as objectives and targets for achievement. The objectives as described below from 2000 to 2020 were closely linked with the federal legislation Omnibus Budget Reconciliation Act (OBRA) (PL 101-239) in 1989 and interagency efforts with the

> **Box 1.3 States and Territories Selected Transition as a NPM**
>
> Alabama, Arizona, Arkansas, California, Connecticut, District of Columbia, Federated States of Micronesia, Florida, Georgia, Guam, Hawaii, Illinois, Indiana, Iowa, Kentucky, Marshall Islands, Maryland, Massachusetts, Michigan, Minnesota, New Jersey, New Mexico, New York, North Dakota, Oklahoma, Oregon, Puerto Rico, Rhode Island, Tennessee, Texas, Utah, Vermont, Virgin Islands, Virginia, Wisconsin, Wyoming
>
> US Department of Health and Human Services, Health Resources and Services Administration's Maternal and Child Health Bureau (n.d.)

Health Resources and Services Administration's Maternal and Child Health Bureau. Over the years as described below, the refinement of objectives for CSHCN and more specifically for HCT has undergone revision.

Healthy People 2000

Based upon Public Law 101-239 OBRA of 1989, the Title V Programs for Children with Special Health Care Needs were now required to develop and implement systems of care for "… the promotion and provision of family-centered, community-based, coordinated care for children with special health care needs;" and "outpatient and community-based services programs for children with special health care needs provided primarily through inpatient institutional care." Additionally, 30% of the funds of the Maternal and Child Health Block Grant Program were to be allocated for CSHCN. These new programmatic requirements resulted in the addition of the following *Healthy People (HP)* Objective in 1990 – 17.20: *Increase to 50 the number of States that have service systems for children with or at risk of chronic and disabling conditions, as required by Public Law 101-239* [51]. This objective reflected the philosophical shift in supporting a different model of care for CSHCN that was more family-focused, accessible, and community-based. This model of care exemplified the changing patterns of the CSHCN lived experience as the advances in medical treatment and interdisciplinary care resulted in improved survival rates.

Healthy People 2010

The *2000 HP* Objective (17.20) was revised with an operational definition that was focused on children rather than the systems of care. This revised HP 2010 objective now read: *Increase the proportion of children with special health care needs who receive their care in family-centered, comprehensive and coordinated systems.* Both the MCHB and Centers for Disease Control and Prevention collaborated in the revision of this objective. The NS-CSHCN and NSCH, funded by the Health Resources and Services Administration's Maternal and Child Health Bureau, were the data sources for measurement of progress as presented in section "National Surveys to Monitor Transition Core Outcome for CSHCN" of this chapter [48].

Healthy People 2020

The transition objective of *HP 2020* was revised again as major efforts were made to only include objectives that could be measured and compared to measurable outcomes. Objectives and sub-objectives of previous *HP* documents were eliminated wherein data sources do not exist that enable measurement of progress and/or achievement in meeting the stated objectives. Transition is one of the sub-objectives (DH-5) of the *HP 2020* Disability and Health Topic Areas and states: *Increase the proportion of youth with special health care needs whose health care provider has discussed transition planning from pediatric to adult health care.* The data source for obtaining measurements of this objective has been the NS-CSHCN, HRSA/ MCHB, and NSCH of CDC. For additional information on data measurement, refer to section "Federal Initiatives to Promote Health Care Transition" as changes have been enacted to obtain more objective measurement data on this objective.

National Surveys to Monitor Transition Core Outcome for CSHCN

In recognition of the necessity to measure progress with achieving the six core outcomes, MCHB embarked upon the development of national surveys to monitor the national- and state-level progress of children's health. The NS-CSHCN was initially designed to track progress with the five of the six core outcomes (Outcomes 2–6 in Table 1.1). NSCH monitored # 1 core outcome (Table 1.1) as well as children's physical and mental health, access to care, and data on the child's community [20]. The evolution of surveys used to collect data on the transition core outcome is described below.

2001 NS-CSHCN Survey Baseline Data of Six Core Outcomes for CSHCN

Monitoring systems were established by MCHB to track the progress with meeting these outcomes during the forthcoming decade (2001–2010) with two new national surveys: the National Survey of Children with Special Health Care Needs

Table 1.1 Core outcomes for CSHCN

No.	Core outcomes	Baseline data 2001 NS-CSHCN and 2001 NHIS meeting outcome criteria
1.	Families of SCHCN will partner in decision-making and will be satisfied with the services that they receive	57.5%
2.	CSHCN will receive coordinated, ongoing, comprehensive care within a medical home	52.6%
3.	Families of CSHCN will have adequate private and/or public insurance to pay for the services that they need	59.6%
4.	Children will be screened early and continuously for special healthcare needs	51.6%
5.	Community-based service systems will be organized so that families can use them easily	74.3%
6.	Youth with special healthcare needs will receive the services necessary to make transitions to adult life, including adult health care, work, and independence	5.8%

McPherson et al. [48, p. 1539]

(NS-CSHCN) and the National Survey of Children's Health (NSCH). NSCH was used to measure progress with Core Outcome 1; NS-CSHCN measured the remaining five core outcomes [48]. The 2001 National Health Interview Survey (NHIS) was employed initially to gather data on Outcome 1.

For each of the outcomes, criteria were operationalized that had to be met to be considered achieved as indicated by survey respondents for youth ages 13–17 years. For Outcome 6, respondents needed to affirm the following two components:

1. Received transition guidance and support

   (a) Doctors discussed changes associated with adulthood.
   (b) Plan developed to address changing needs.
   (c) Transfer of care to adult providers discussed.

2. Received vocational/career training

As noted in the baseline data gathered for the six core outcomes, Outcome 6 was the least achieved of all of the outcomes (Table 1.1).

Table 1.2 presents the findings associated with the components of the transition core outcome reported from the 2001 NS-CSHCN Survey. Less than 20% (15.3%) of respondents indicated having received guidance as described in component 1; 25.5% replied that vocational/career training had been received (Table 1.2).

Additional analysis of this data was reported as associated with race/ethnicity. There were significant differences by race/ethnicity of those who reported doctors discussed changes associated with adulthood. Just 31.6% of Hispanic respondents reported these discussions with their physicians compared to 52.1% non-Hispanic whites, 49.9% non-Hispanic blacks, and 49.9% non-Hispanic other race/ethnicity ($p = .00016$) [42]. Other ethnic/racial significant differences in patterns of responses were noted as well. When asked if discussion had ensued about the transfer to adult

Table 1.2 Transition core outcome and components based on the 2001 NS-CSHCN Survey

	Percent achieved
YSCHN achieved transition core outcome	5.8%
Components	
Received guidance pertaining to healthcare aspects of transition	15.3%
Transfer of care to adult providers discussed	41.8%
Doctors discussed changes associated with adulthood	50%
Plan developed to address changing needs	59.3%
Received vocational/career training	25.5%

McPherson et al. [48]

providers, non-Hispanic blacks (38.1%) and non-Hispanic whites (40.6%) differed significantly from Hispanics (56.4%) and non-Hispanic others (58.8%) ($p = .03$).

The percentage of older adolescents (16–17 years) (19.5%) reporting affirmatively to meeting the transition core outcome was significantly higher than for younger adolescents (13–15 years) (12.9%) ($p = .001$). Significant differences were reported for adolescents meeting the transition core outcome who reported having a medical home (20.1%) compared to those who did not (11.4%) ($p = .000$) [42].

2005–2006 NS-CSHCN Survey Findings

Data were gathered again with the 2005–2006 NS-CSHCN Survey to assess the extent to which progress had been achieved with the six core outcomes. Core Outcome 6 was measured differently in the 2005–2006 Survey. There were variations in the item measuring the transition outcome. The vocational and career training component was excluded and discussion about health insurance coverage was added [43]. Queries were added about encouraging the youth to self-manage and assume responsibility for their care needs, and future planning for health needs as an adult was explicated. As with the earlier 2001 NS-CSHCN Survey, all elements had to be met to affirm the youth had received transition guidance and support: (a) transfer of care to adult providers; (b) doctors discussed changes associated with adulthood; (c) changes with insurance coverage as an adult; and (d) assumption of self-management responsibilities encouraged. Findings associated with the transition outcomes were as presented in Table 1.3.

As with the earlier national survey, NS-CSHCN, the transition core outcome lagged behind the other CSHCN core outcomes. However, comparisons between the earlier 2001 NS-CSHCN and 2005–2006 NS-CSHCN are difficult to make as the items were changed during the interim period of time. Of note, significant disparities were again found among groups surveyed. Findings revealed that 47.6% of non-Hispanic white youth, ages 12–17, attained the transition core outcome compared to 28.7% non-Hispanic black youth and 26.3% Hispanic youth. The odds of

Table 1.3 Transition core outcome based on 2005–2006 NS-CSHCN Survey

	Percent achieved
YSCHN achieved transition core outcome	41%
Components	
Transfer of care to adult providers	42%
Doctors discussed changes associated with adulthood	62%
Changes with insurance coverage as an adult	34%
Assumption of self-management responsibilities encouraged	78%

Lotstein et al. [43]

not achieving the transition core outcome was 1.5 and 1.43 times greater ($p \leq .05$) for non-Hispanic black and Hispanic youth, respectively [43, 44]. A number of factors were identified as contributory to these disparities, which included access to health insurance, living in low-resourced communities, and sociocultural factors such as educational level and attitudes toward future planning and healthcare providers.

2016 National Survey of Children's Health Findings on Healthcare Transition Planning

In 2016, the National Survey of Children's Health (NSCH) was conducted that gathered data from a representative national survey of 50, 212 children and youth, 0–17 years, of whom 20, 708 were ages 12–17. The 2016 NSCH integrated for the first time previous NSCH and National Survey of Children with Special Health Care Needs (NS-CSHCN). This survey was designed to collect comprehensive data on children's and youth's physical and mental health, demographic data including parents/caregivers and the child's social network (i.e., school and community) [20]. Items included queries pertaining to children and youth with special healthcare needs such as health insurance, access to care, and chronic care management.

Data on the progress of facilitating the HCT of adolescents with/without SHCN were gathered as well. Parents/caregivers of adolescents ages 12–17 were asked questions that corresponded with the NPM and the 2011 Clinical Report guidelines [38]. The measure of transition planning as reported in the 2016 NSCH is a composite score based on the four survey items: (a) speaking privately with the provider during the preventive care visit; (b) transfer of care to adult provider; (c) changes associated age 18 (in some states, considered the age of majority); and (d) self-management instruction. Items c and d were combined for data analysis purposes as "provider active work with youth" [38, p. 3]. The scoring of youth as receiving HCT services was based upon affirmative responses to all three items. Findings revealed 17% of YSHCN and 14% of youth without SHCN received all elements of

HCT. Higher percentage of YSHCN (23%) and those without SHCN (18%) ages 15–17 received HCT services as compared to those age 12–14 years. Those who reported receiving care coordination and written care plan were more likely to report having received HCT services [38]. As the NSCH findings demonstrate, much work is needed to ensure that all youth receive the HCT services needed to facilitate their uninterrupted transfer of care to adult services and to have them well prepared to function as informed, literate consumers of health care and to function independently as possible in managing their own healthcare needs.

Federal Initiatives to Promote Healthcare Transition

Beginning in the late 1990s, the Health Resources and Services Administration's Maternal and Child Health Bureau allocated funding to support the development of community-based HCT demonstration projects and national resource centers. This section provides an overview of those efforts that have been undertaken for the past two decades.

Healthy and Ready to Work

In the mid-1990s the Division of Children with Special Health Care Needs, Maternal and Child Health Bureau, launched a national initiative in HCT, entitled *Healthy and Ready to Work (HRTW)*. The initial effort was directed to funding innovative community-based pilot programs in HCT. Each of the funded projects was involved with outreach training for interdisciplinary colleagues from health and non-health organizations, provision of technical assistance to interagency providers, and development of HCT resources for dissemination to diverse constituents that included adolescents with SHCN, families, service providers, and policymakers. Each of the projects was unique in their goals and objectives although they shared commonalities of purpose. Two cycles of funding were available for these early pilot projects. It was during this time funding was allocated for a national HCT resource center. This first center, *Healthy and Ready to Work (HRTW) National Center*, was established in 2001 and was the precursor resource center of *Got Transition*.

National Resource Center for HCT: *Got Transition*

Got Transition serves as a comprehensive HCT resource center funded by the Maternal and Child Health Bureau. Its website contains resources for youth and families, researchers and policymakers, and healthcare providers. *Got Transition* staff are active in the development and dissemination of HCT resources, compiling a repository of HCT evidence and research conducted and providing technical assistance to systems of care in developing HCT service models. *Got Transition* in conjunction with the Maternal and Child Health Bureau has undertaken policymaking efforts to promote the development of HCT services within the pediatric systems of health care.

Of relevance to the development and implementation of HCT services in healthcare service setting is a guideline template to provide guidance in the elemental components of establishing a model of care. This guideline template is referred to as the Six Core Elements of Transition 2.0 (Got Transition, 2014). The Sixth Core Elements include (a) the establishment of a HCT policy that specifies the benchmarks of services provided; (b) establishment of a monitoring system that enables tracking of the youth's and young adult's progress in achieving HCT predetermined goals; (c) use of a transition readiness assessment to monitor acquisition of HCT skills and knowledge; (d) development, implementation, and evaluation of HCT adolescent-centered plan that is based upon individualized needs focused on the transfer of care process; and (e) initiation of the transfer process that includes the confirmation that care has been transferred and established with adult providers.

Development of the HCT Field of Science and Practice

Healthcare Transition Research Consortium

In 2008, a group of colleagues, the early "pioneers" in the field of HCT, understood the wisdom and necessity of networking together and creating a forum wherein their work, questions, and experiences could be shared. These early visionaries were led by Maria E. Diaz-Gonzalez de Ferris, MD, MPH, PhD, and David L. Wood, MD, MPH, and under their leadership established the Health Care Transition Research Consortium (HCTRC). Initially, conference calls were scheduled to informally share information and provide updates pertaining to research and practice efforts. Concomitantly, small gatherings were held at the University of North Carolina, Chapel Hill, to discuss HCT topics of interest and current research projects underway.

Four year later, in 2012 HCTRC partnered with the Baylor College of Medicine and Texas Children's Hospital that had been hosting, under the leadership of Dr. Albert Hergenroeder, the annual HCT conference entitled *Chronic Illness and Disability Conference: Transition from Pediatric to Adult-Based Care* since 1999. That partnership enabled the hosting of the annual HCTRC Research Symposium held in conjunction with the annual Transition from Pediatric to Adult-Based Care conference. The symposium draws well-known international and national speakers to present their research and network with one another. It is the only research forum in the United States devoted solely to HCT. Another research forum, inspired in part by the HCTRC Research Symposium, has now been hosted in Switzerland.

Under the leadership of HCTRC members, a number of endeavors have been undertaken to promote the relevancy and importance of HCT as well as direct attention to this field of practice and research. Under the editorship of Drs. Wood, Ferris, and John Reiss, (inaugural members of HCTRC and early HCT "pioneers") an entire issue entitled *Youth Health Care Transition* was published in the *International Journal of Child and Adolescent Health*. This publication was a landmark development as it was the first time that an entire issue had been published on the topic of HCT which was composed of 16 review and research articles.

Other articles were published by the HCTRC Consortium, which included HCTRC HCT model to guide practice and research [11] and Delphi survey to identify HCT outcomes [24]. Each year HCTRC sponsors a Special Interest Group, Health Care Transition, and Self-Management at the annual Pediatric Academic Societies meetings. Other ongoing activities include monthly conference calls involving Consortium members nationally and internationally that enable them to share their work, updates, and pending events of interests and information about the annual HCTRC Research Symposium.

This consortium has done much to foster the development of the field of practice and research through these activities. HCTRC has been the sole network dedicated solely to a number of efforts to realize its mission. HCTRC has been engaged in promoting dissemination of research currently produced, facilitating updates on current developments in the field of HCT as it pertains to legislative, policymaking, and research initiatives and enabling networking among colleagues involved with HCT research, quality improvement, and scholarly efforts.

State of Research, Clinical Practice, and Beyond

In 2004, the first comprehensive narrative HCT review of literature was published. This early review covered a span of 21 years from 1982 to 2003 and included 43 studies. These early studies lacked rigorous designs and methodology. The research designs were primarily descriptive; none of the studies included comparison or control groups. None of the studies reported the use of tools with needed psychometric measurements of validity and reliability. The topical foci of studies of this review examined adolescent and parental HCT needs, HCT barriers, and transfer criteria. However, these studies represented the emerging field of practice and science and provided early guidance and recommendations for subsequent practice and research [10].

Since that early narrative review, the volume and quality of research conducted are apparent with the publication of HCT systematic reviews that provide critical analyses of HCT studies on selected topics (i.e., examination and analysis of HCT outcomes). A recent review of systematic reviews reported a total of 37 systematic reviews involving 71 studies that met eligibility criteria that have been conducted to date since 2004 [27].

Major findings of the review reported the following: More than half of the reviews have been published since 2014. Quantitative synthesis was lacking in all but one of these reviews; one review reported meta-analysis of four studies within the larger review that was qualitatively focused [63]. Using the AMSTAR criteria for assessment of the quality of the reviews, 12 of the 37 studies were considered to be high-quality reviews [65]. Four randomized control trials were reported in reviews. The reviews represented divergent areas of focus. Although 20 of the 37 were not diagnostic focused, of those that were, type 1 diabetes was the focus of 7 reviews, and 2 were conducted on mental health. Exploration of transition interventions was conducted in 14 reviews. As noted, 14 (19.7%) of the 71 studies addressed interventions associated with adult care following the transfer of care.

The limitations evident in the reviews were the variability in the quality of the reviews. Several components considered essential in quality reviews were missing such as publication bias, quality assessment metrics of studies reviewed. Just one of the reviews was registered in PROSPERO, a website that provides a listing and status report of systematic reviews being conducted.

A recent systematic review with updated examination of HCT outcomes following an earlier systematic review was conducted by the members of the authoring team with studies published between May 2016 and December 2018 [25, 62]. Nineteen studies were included in this review. Examination of the HCT interventions was based upon the 2018 AAP/AAFP/ACP Clinical Report Guidelines [69]. The studies included in this review reflected an international perspective as five (26%) were conducted in the United States, four in Australia, three in Canada, and two in the Netherlands. As reported in the Hart et al. review [27], the most frequently cited condition reported was type 1 diabetes. Other chronic conditions reported were congenital heart disease, inflammatory bowel disease, juvenile idiopathic arthritis, and kidney transplants. The Triple Aim framework was used to report outcomes [70]. The following positive outcomes were reported according to this framework: population (11; 65%); patient experience (1; 5%); and utilization of care (6; 60%). All studies reported the transfer of care assistance; nearly all referred to one transition planning activity (i.e., patient education; medical summary) and integration into adult care (i.e., follow-up on first appointment with adult provider).

The Effective Public Health Practice Project Quality Assessment Tool for Quantitative Studies to assess the quality of studies is included in the review [68]. Study strengths were reported as follows: two studies as strong (11%); ten studies as moderate (53%) and seven as weak (37%). Noteworthily, 74% of the studies did not report the psychometrics of the tools used for measurement; 58% did not have sufficient controls for confounding variables (i.e., lack of randomization).

As evident with the growing body of HCT literature, the studies being reported are contributing to an improved understanding of the phenomenon of HCT. As this body of evidence evolves, issues as to the design and implementation of strategies that effect positive biopsychosocial and health outcomes for adolescents and young adults with chronic conditions will be better understood. As reported in the most current reviews of the literature, the science is slowly emerging that will assist with the development of service models that improve outcomes of care, are cost-effective, and meet with the satisfaction of the consumers who use them [70].

Conclusion

This chapter provided an overview of the development of the healthcare transition field of practice and science since its initial emergence as a service need for the growing population of adolescents and young adults with chronic conditions and disabilities 30 years ago. As has been detailed in this chapter, government investment, visionary leadership, and the advocacy and support of professional medical associations were pivotal agents of change in providing the impetus needed in fostering the growth of this important area of practice and research. As delineated in this chapter, the past efforts recorded here have led to the steady movement forward in shaping new and innovative models of service that will better serve this population of youth and young adults.

References

1. Agrawal R, Hall M, Cohen E, et al. Trends in health care spending for children in medicaid with high resource use. Pediatrics. 2016;138(4):e20160682. https://doi.org/10.1542/peds.2016-0682.
2. American Academy of Pediatrics. Age limits of pediatrics. J Pediatr. 1938;13(127):266.
3. American Academy of Pediatrics. Council on Child Health Age limits of pediatrics. Pediatrics. 1972;49(3):463.
4. American Academy of Pediatrics. Council on Child and Adolescent Health: age limits of pediatrics. Pediatrics. 1988;81(5):736.
5. American Academy of Pediatrics (AAP), American Academy of Family Physicians (AAFP) and American College of Physicians (ACP). American Society of Internal Medicine A consensus statement on health care transitions for young adults with special health care needs. Pediatrics. 2002;110(6 Pt 2):1304–6.
6. American Academy of Pediatrics, Committee on Children with Disabilities and Committee on Adolescence. Transition of care provided for adolescents with special health care needs. Pediatrics. 1996;98(6 Pt 1):1203–6.
7. American Academy of Pediatrics, American Academy of Family Physicians, American College of Physicians, Transitions Clinical Report Authoring Group, Cooley WC, Sagerman PJ. Supporting the health care transition from adolescence to adulthood in the medical home. Pediatrics. 2011;128(1):182–200. https://doi.org/10.1542/peds.2011-0969. Epub 2011 Jun 27. PubMed PMID: 21708806.
8. Arnett JJ. Emerging adulthood. A theory of development from the late teens through the twenties. Am Psychol. 2000;55(5):469–80.
9. Association of Maternal and Child Health Programs. Celebrating the legacy, shaping the future: 75 years of state and federal partnership to improve maternal and child health. Crystal City: Author; 2010. Retrieved on 19 Jan 2020 from: http://www.amchp.org/AboutTitleV/Documents/Celebrating-the-Legacy.pdf.
10. Betz CL. Transition of adolescents with special health care needs: review and analysis of the literature. Issues Compr Pediatr Nurs. 2004;27:179–240.
11. Betz CL, Ferris ME, Woodward JF, Okumura M, Jan S, Wood DL, authoring group for the Health Care Transition Research Consortium. The health care transition research consortium health care transition model: a framework for research and practice. J Pediatr Rehabil Med. 2014;7:3–15. https://doi.org/10.3233/PRM-140277.

12. Blum RW. Transition to adult health care: setting the stage. J Adolesc Health. 1995;17:3–5. https://doi.org/10.1016/1054-139X(95)00073-2.

13. Blum RW, Garell D, Hodgman CH, Jorissen TW, Okinow NA, Orr DP, Slap GB. Transition from child-centered to adult health-care systems for adolescents with chronic conditions. A position paper of the Society for Adolescent Medicine. J Adolesc Health. 1993;14(7):570–6.

14. Chaturvedi S, DeBaun M. Evolution of sickle cell disease from a life-threatening disease of children to a chronic disease of adults: the last 40 years. Am J Hematol. 2016;91(1):5–14. https://doi.org/10.1002/ajh.24235.

15. Chonat S, Quinn C, Malik P, Tisdale J. Current standards of care and long term outcomes for thalassemia and sickle cell disease. In: Gene and cell therapies for beta-globinopathies, 1013; 2017. p. 905–87. https://doi.org/10.1007/978-1-4939-7299-9_3.

16. Clarizia NA, Chahal N, Manlhiot C, Kilburn J, Redington AN, McCrindle BW. Transition to adult health care for adolescents and young adults with congenital heart disease: perspectives of the patient, parent and health care provider. Can J Cardiol. 2009;25(9):e317–22.

17. Cohen E, Kuo DZ, Agrawal R, et al. Children with medical complexity: an emerging population for clinical and research initiatives. Pediatrics. 2011;127(3):529–38. https://doi.org/10.1542/peds.2010-0910.

18. Cystic Fibrosis Foundation. Cystic fibrosis foundation patient registry highlights. 2017. Retrieved on 10 Jan 2020 from: https://www.cff.org/Research/Researcher-Resources/Patient-Registry/2017-Cystic-Fibrosis-Foundation-Patient-Registry-Highlights.pdf.

19. Cystic Fibrosis Trust. UK CF Registry at-a-glance report 2017 [online] Cystic Fibrosis Trust. 2018. Retrieved on 11 Jan 2020 from: https://www.cysticfibrosis.org.uk/the-work-we-do/uk-cf-registry/reporting-and-resources/ata-glance-report-2017.

20. Data Resource Center for Child and Adolescent Health. National survey of children's health. n.d. Retrieved on 6 Feb 2020 from: https://www.childhealthdata.org/learn-about-the-nsch/NSCH.

21. De Boeck K. Cystic fibrosis in the year 2020: a disease with a new face. Acta Paediatr. 2020; https://doi.org/10.1111/apa.15155.

22. Dow-Edwards D, MacMaster F, Peterson B, Niesink R, Andersen S, Braams B. Experience during adolescence shapes brain development: from synapses and networks to normal and pathological behavior. Neurotoxicol Teratol. 2019;76:106834. https://doi.org/10.1016/j.ntt.2019.106834.

23. Eagle M, Baudouin S, Chandler C, Giddings D, Bullock R, Bushby K. Survival in Duchenne muscular dystrophy: improvements in life expectancy since 1967 and the impact of home nocturnal ventilation. Neuromuscul Disord. 2002;12(10):926–9. https://doi.org/10.1016/s0960-8966(02)00140-2.

24. Fair C, Cuttance J, Sharma N, Maslow G, Wiener L, Betz CL, Porter J, McLaughlin S, Gilleland-Marchak J, Renwick A, Naranjo D, Jan S, Javalkar K, Ferris M, for the International and Interdisciplinary Health Care Transition Research Consortium. International and interdisciplinary identification of health care transition outcomes. JAMA Pediatr. Published online 30 Nov 2015. 2015; https://doi.org/10.1001/jamapediatrics.2016.3168.

25. Gabriel P, McManus M, Rogers K, White P. Outcome evidence for structured pediatric to adult health care transition interventions: a systematic review. J Pediatr. 2017;188:263–269. e15. https://doi.org/10.1016/j.jpeds.2017.05.066. Epub 2017 Jun 28. Review. PubMed PMID: 28668449.

26. Hardin AP, Hackell JM. Committee on Practice and Ambulatory Medicine. Pediatrics. 2017;140(3):e20172151. https://doi.org/10.1542/peds.2017-2151.

27. Hart LC, Patel-Nguyen SV, Merkley MG, Jonas DE. An evidence map for interventions addressing transition from pediatric to adult care: a systematic review of systematic reviews. J Pediatr Nurs. 2019;48:18–34. https://doi.org/10.1016/j.pedn.2019.05.015. Epub 2019 Jun 17. Review. PubMed PMID: 31220801.

28. Hunt G, Poulton A. Open spina bifida: a complete cohort reviewed 25 years after closure. Dev Med Child Neurol. 1995;37(1):19–29. https://doi.org/10.1111/j.1469-8749.1995.tb11929.x.

29. Hutchins VL, McPherson M. National agenda for children with special health needs: social policy for the 1990s through the 21st century. Am Psychol. 1991;46(2):141–3. https://doi.org/1 0.1037//0003-066x.46.2.141.

30. Ireys HT, Nelson RP. New federal policy for children with special health care needs: implications for pediatricians. Pediatrics. 1992;90(3):321–7.

31. Ireys HT, Hauck RJ, Perrin JM. Variability among state Crippled Children's Service programs: pluralism thrives. Am J Public Health. 1985;75(4):375–81. https://doi.org/10.2105/ajph.75.4.375.

32. Kieny P, Chollet S, Delalande P, Le Fort M, Magot A, Pereon Y, Perrouin VB. Evolution of life expectancy of patients with Duchenne muscular dystrophy at AFM Yolaine de Kepper centre between 1981 and 2011. Ann Phys Rehabil Med. 2013;56(6):443–54. https://doi.org/10.1016/j.rehab.2013.06.002.

33. Kogan M, Dykton C, Hirai A, Strickland B, Bethell C, Naqvi I, et al. A new performance measurement system for maternal and child health in the United States. Matern Child Health J. 2015;19(5):945–57. https://doi.org/10.1007/s10995-015-1739-5.

34. Koop CE. Introductory remarks. In: McGrab P, Millar H, editors. Surgeon general's conference. Growing up and getting medical care: youth with special health care needs. Washington, DC: National Center for Networking Community Based Services, Georgetown University Child Development Center; 1989. Retrieved on 8 Jan 2020 from: https://profiles.nlm.nih.gov/spotlight/nn/catalog/nlm:nlmuid-101584932X870-doc.

35. Kuo DZ, Cohen E, Agrawal R, Berry JG, Casey PH. MDA national profile of caregiver challenges among more medically complex children with special health care needs. Arch Pediatr Adolesc Med. 2011;165(11):1020–6. https://doi.org/10.1001/archpediatrics.2011.172.

36. Kuo DZ, Melguizo-Castro M, Goudie A, Nick TG, Robbins JM, Casey PH. Variation in child health care utilization by medical complexity. Matern Child Health J. 2015;19(1):40–8. https://doi.org/10.1007/s10995-014-1493-0.

37. Laurence K. Occasional survey. Lancet. 1974;1(7852):301–4. https://doi.org/10.1016/s0140-6736(74)92606-3.

38. Lebrun-Harris LA, McManus MA, Ilango SM, et al. Transition planning among US youth with and without special health care needs. Pediatrics. 2018;142(4):e20180194.

39. Lipkin P, Okamoto J, the Council on Children with Disabilities and Council on School Health. The Individuals With Disabilities Education Act (IDEA) for children with special educational needs. Pediatrics. 2015;136(6):e1650–62. https://doi.org/10.1542/peds.2015-3409.

40. Litt IF. Age limits of pediatrics, American Academy of Pediatrics, Council on Child Health, Pediatrics, 1972;49:463. Pediatrics. 1998;102(1 Pt 2):249–50.

41. Lorber J. Results of treatment of myelomeningocele. An analysis of 524 unselected cases, with special reference to possible selection for treatment. Dev Med Child Neurol, 1973. 1971;13(3):279–303.

42. Lotstein DS, McPherson M, Strickland B, Newacheck PW. Transition planning for youth with special health care needs: results from the national survey of children with special health care needs. Pediatrics. 2005;115(6):1562–8. https://doi.org/10.1542/peds.2004-1262.

43. Lotstein DS, Ghandour R, Cash A, McGuire E, Strickland B, Newacheck P. Planning for health care transitions: results from the 2005-2006 National Survey of Children with Special Health Care Needs. Pediatrics. 2009;123(1):e145–52. https://doi.org/10.1542/peds.2008-1298. PubMed PMID: 19117836.

44. Lotstein DS, Kuo AA, Strickland B, Tait F. The transition to adult health care for youth with special health care needs: do racial and ethnic disparities exist? Pediatrics. 2010;126(3):S129–36. https://doi.org/10.1542/peds.2010-1466F.

45. McGrab P, Millar H, eds. Executive summary In: Surgeon General's Conference. Growing up and getting medical care: youth with special health care needs. Washington, DC: National Center for Networking Community Based Services, Georgetown University Child Development Center; 1989. Retrieved on 8 Jan 2020 from: https://profiles.nlm.nih.gov/spotlight/nn/catalog/nlm:nlmuid-101584932X870-doc

46. McLaughlin J, Shurtleff D, Lamers J, Stuntz J, Hayden P, Kropp R. Influence of prognosis on decisions regarding the care of newborns with myelodysplasia. NEJM. 1985;312(25):1589–94. https://doi.org/10.1056/NEJM198506203122501.

47. McManus M, White P. Transition to adult health care services for young adults with chronic medical illness and psychiatric comorbidity. Child Adolesc Psychiatr Clin N Am. 2017;26(2):367–80. PubMed PMID: 28314461.

48. McPherson M, Weissman G, Strickland BB, van Dyck PC, Blumberg SJ, Newacheck PW. Implementing community-based systems of services for children and youths with special health care needs: how well are we doing? Pediatrics. 2004;113(5 Suppl):1538–44.

49. National Association of Pediatric Nurse Practitioners (NAPNAP). NAPNAP Position statement on age parameters for pediatric nurse practitioner practice. 2008. Retrieved on 28 Jan 2012 from http://download.journals.elsevierhealth.com/pdfs/journals/0891-5245/PIIS0891524508000552.pdf.

50. National Center for Health Statistics. Healthy People 2000 Review, 1995-1996. Hyattsville, Maryland: Public Health Service. 1996.

51. National Center for Health Statistics. Healthy people 2000 final review. Hyattsville: Public Health Service; 2001.

52. National Center for Health Statistics. Healthy people 2000 progress review: diabetes and chronic disabling conditions. Retrieved on 10 Feb 2020 from: https://www.cdc.gov/nchs/data/hp2000/diabetes/17obj.pdf.

53. Nehring WN, Betz CL, Lobo ML. Uncharted territory: systematic review of providers' roles, understanding and views pertaining to health care transition. J Pediatr Nurs. 2015;30(5):732–47. https://doi.org/10.1016/j.pedn.2015.05.030.

54. Oakeshott P, Poulton A, Hunt G. Reid F Expectation of life and unexpected death in open spina bifida: a 40-year complete, non-selective, longitudinal cohort study. Dev Med Child Neurol. 2009;52(8):749–53. https://doi.org/10.1111/j.1469-8749.2009.03543.x.

55. Oakeshott P, Poulton A, Hunt G, Reid F. Walking and living independently with spina bifida: a 50-year prospective cohort study. Dev Med Child Neurol. 2019;61(10):1202–7. https://doi.org/10.1111/dmcn.14168.

56. Office of Disease Prevention and Health Promotion. Healthy people 2020 disability and health, barriers to health care, DH-5. 2010. Retrieved on 7 Feb 2020 from : https://www.healthypeople.gov/2020/topics-objectives/topic/disability-and-health/objectives

57. Okumura MJ, Kerr EA, Cabana MD, Davis MM, Demonner S, Heisler M. Physician views on barriers to primary care for young adults with childhood-onset chronic disease. Pediatrics. 2010;125(4):e748–54.

58. Perrin JM, Bloom SR, Gortmaker SL. The increase of childhood chronic conditions in the United States. JAMA. 2007;297:2755–9.

59. Quinn C, Rogers Z, McCavit T, Buchanan G. Improved survival of children and adolescents with sickle cell disease. Blood. 2010;115(17):3447–52. https://doi.org/10.1182/blood-2009-07-233700.

60. Roebroeck ME, Jahnsen R, Carona C, Kent RM, Chamberlain MA. Adult outcomes and lifespan issues for people with childhood-onset physical disability. Dev Med Child Neurol. 2009;51(8):670–8.

61. Rosen D. Between two worlds: bridging the cultures of child health and adult medicine. J Adolesc Health. 1995;17:10–6. https://doi.org/10.1016/1054-139X(95)00077-6.

62. Schmidt A, Ilango SM, McManus MA, Rogers KK, White PH. Outcomes of pediatric to adult health care transition interventions: an updated systematic review. J Pediatr Nurs. 2020;51:92–107. https://doi.org/10.1016/j.pedn.2020.01.002. [Epub ahead of print] Review. PubMed PMID: 31981969.

63. Schultz A, Smaldone A. Components of interventions that improve transitions to adult care for adolescents with type 1 diabetes. J Adolesc Health. 2017;60(2):133–46. https://doi.org/10.1016/j.jadohealth.2016.10.002.

64. Scott R. Health care priority and sickle cell anemia. JAMA. 1970;214(4):731–4.

65. Shea BJ, Hamel C, Wells GA, Bouter LM, Kristjansson E, Grimshaw J, et al. AMSTAR is a reliable and valid measurement tool to assess the methodological quality of systematic reviews. J Clin Epidemiol. 2009;62(10):1013–20.
66. Simmonds N. Ageing in cystic fibrosis and long-term survival. Paediatr Respir Rev. 2013;14(1):6–9. https://doi.org/10.1016/j.prrv.2013.01.007.
67. Summary of conference recommendations. J Adolesc Health. 1995;17:6–9. https://doi.org/10.1016/1054-139X(95)00074-3.
68. Thomas BH, Ciliska D, Dobbins M, Micucci S. A process for systematically reviewing the literature: providing the research evidence for public health nursing interventions. Worldviews Evid-Based Nurs. 2004;1(3):176–84.
69. White PH, Cooley WC, Transitions Clinical Report Authoring Group, American Academy of Pediatrics, American Academy of Family Physicians, American College of Physicians. Supporting the health care transition from adolescence to adulthood in the medical home. Pediatrics. 2018;142(5):e20182587. (2019). Pediatrics, 143(2). https://doi.org/10.1542/peds.2018-3610.
70. Whittington JW, Nolan K, Lewis N, Torres T. Pursuing the triple aim: the first 7 years. Milbank Q. 2015;93(2):263–300. https://doi.org/10.1111/1468-0009.12122.

Chapter 2
Transition Research: Approaches to Measurement and Outcomes

Cory Powers and Cynthia D. Brown

Introduction

In 1989, the Surgeon General of the United States, C. Everett Koop, MD, convened a conference to address the needs of the growing population of adolescents and young adults (AYA) with special healthcare needs as they transitioned from pediatric to adult health care [1]. In this report, it was noted that there was a lack of research to define optimal landmarks and timing of transition readiness. In addition, the research infrastructure did not exist to examine the outcomes after transition [1]. Over the ensuing decades, and as health care for AYA improved, the number of individuals entering the adult healthcare system with chronic illness has continued to increase. In the most recent National Survey of Children's Health (NSCH) performed in 2017–2018, 13.6 million children (18.5%) were identified as having a special healthcare need defined as "increased risk for a chronic physical, developmental, behavioral, or emotional condition and who also require health and related services of a type or amount beyond that required by children generally." Moreover, almost 25% of households had more than one child with special healthcare needs [2]. Despite more than three decades since the original Surgeon General's call to action on transition needs, most youth fail to have appropriate transition support. In the NSCH, only 17% of youth with special healthcare needs and 14% of youth without

C. Powers
Departments of Internal Medicine and Pediatrics, Indiana University School of Medicine, Indianapolis, IN, USA
e-mail: compower@iupui.edu

C. D. Brown (✉)
Division of Pulmonary, Critical Care, Occupational, and Sleep Medicine, Indiana University School of Medicine, Indianapolis, IN, USA
e-mail: cyndbrow@iu.edu

© Springer Nature Switzerland AG 2021
C. D. Brown, E. Crowley (eds.), *Transitioning Care from Pediatric to Adult Pulmonology*, Respiratory Medicine,
https://doi.org/10.1007/978-3-030-68688-8_2

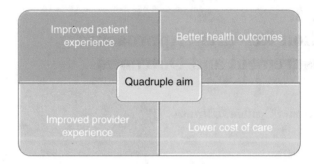

Fig. 2.1 Quadruple aim for quality improvement in health care. The goal of the quadruple aim is to improve quality of care by improving patient experience, improving provider experience, providing better health outcomes, and lowering cost of care. (Adapted from Bodenheimer and Sinsky [4])

special healthcare needs reported receiving transition services from their healthcare provider (HCP) [3]. In addition, research into best practices and outcomes around transition continue to be lacking. This review will outline the current state of knowledge regarding measurement of transition readiness in AYA and outcomes of transition framed in the context of the quadruple aim for quality improvement: improving patient experience, improving health outcomes, lowering cost of care, and improving provider experience (Fig. 2.1) [4]. The review will also highlight ongoing areas of need for a future research agenda for AYA transitioning to adult care.

Overview of Qualitative Research in Transition Medicine

Qualitative research relies on the systematic collection and analysis of information derived from observation or interviews [5]. For many individuals in the medical sciences, the performance and interpretation of qualitative materials have been difficult to conceptualize and integrate into the research portfolio. Qualitative research is more often utilized in the social sciences and, when considering transition practices, can be utilized to help understand patient, family, and provider values and experiences at the time of transition from pediatric to adult care. Understanding the tools used in qualitative research can be important for assessing quality of care and help explain variations in care provision. Characteristics of qualitative research compared to quantitative research are outlined in Fig. 2.2. Qualitative research has the advantages of taking an in-depth, personalized assessment of a problem in a holistic manner. Some of the common scenarios when qualitative methods are applied include sensitive topics of research, unexplored areas of research, need to understand the lived experience of individuals, and in-depth assessment of a program or intervention [6]. Qualitative methods can also be combined with quantitative assessments in a mixed-methods approach to further inform decision-making. Qualitative research theory is detailed and is the basis of significant study beyond the scope of this review.

Fig. 2.2 Comparison of qualitative and quantitative research. (Adapted from Padgett [6])

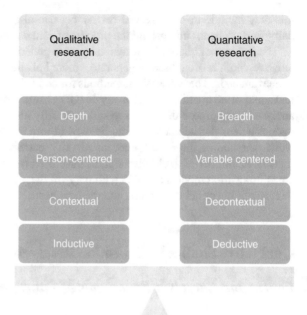

The most commonly used tools in qualitative research include interviewing, observation, and analysis of documents [5]. Interview-based methods can be semi-structured or in-depth and can be done one-on-one or in focus groups. Before engaging in interview-based methods, the interviewer should be trained in the conduct of these interviews within the context of qualitative research in order to maximize data collection and minimize bias. In a semi-structured interview, the researcher develops a topic guide with a loose structure of open-ended questions. While the researcher desires to cover the proposed questions, there is flexibility to allow the researcher to follow a topic of interest as it comes up in the interview. The purpose of a semi-structured interview is often to delve into an individual's experiences and attitudes. In a focus group, a trained moderator leads the interview process in a group of about ten individuals, although the size of the group may vary based upon the question. A focus group provides the benefit of learning from shared experiences within the group and allows collection of a larger amount of data over time when compared to one-on-one interviews.

Observational methods are often utilized for assessment of a practice, such as delivery of care or in an organizational setting. Observation can also be used to evaluate the behavior of individuals in different situations rather than relying on interview reports alone. To perform qualitative observational research, the researcher needs to determine the level of participation prior to engaging in the research and also consider how the act of observation may change behavior, a phenomenon known as reactivity [6]. Finally, the narrative review of previously collected documents is another common way of performing qualitative research. In health care, this may include medical record review but can also include documents used in daily work to better understand the process of care delivery.

The purpose of qualitative research is not to generate numeric data; rather qualitative research is often used to generate a more holistic overview of a topic through textual analysis. There are robust methods for codifying and analyzing the collected texts, and often qualitative data analysis (QDA) software is used to standardize the analysis. The purpose of QDA is to systematically identify common themes or categories across participants that can be used in turn to develop a theoretical framework that allows the investigator to identify patterns and develop explanatory models. A number of qualitative studies have been performed over the years in the area of transition models for AYA with many of these focusing on the experience of the patient, his or her caregivers, and the healthcare providers.

Qualitative Studies in Transition Research

Patient and Caregiver Experience of Transition

Numerous qualitative studies have evaluated the experiences of AYA and their caregivers during the transition from pediatric to adult healthcare services in a variety of disease processes. Regarding transition, the most commonly studied diseases include type 1 diabetes mellitus, congenital heart disease, cystic fibrosis, mental health, and complex healthcare needs such as autism spectrum disorders [7–12]. A variety of methods were utilized including semi-structured interviews and focus groups. Common themes that arise across multiple studies include preparation for transition and transfer, gaining independence and responsibility, and concerns about changing relationships and unfamiliar cultures [8, 9]. Regarding transition preparation and transfer, patients across several studies felt that age alone should not signal a readiness for transition and that transition readiness should be the deciding factor regardless of age [8, 9, 13]. Practices regarding transition preparation and readiness are highly variable among clinics and specialties. In many clinics, healthcare providers (HCPs) acknowledged that transition and transfer of care occur without formalized policies and education, primarily related to lack of time and resources [8]. Abrupt transitions were viewed more negatively by AYA, leading to feelings of abandonment and resentment. Also, transferring care at times that coincided with transitions in other aspects of life (illness, graduation, moving away from home, etc.) was viewed by AYA as more stressful [9]. Conversely, transition was typically felt by AYA as a natural progression in their level of responsibility and independence. Most AYA acknowledged that transition into adult care assumed that the individual, rather than the parent, would be the primary person responsible for decision-making regarding health care. For some, transition was viewed as an important milestone in their care and lives; for others, the anxiety associated with transition felt overwhelming. AYA also expressed sadness about leaving long-standing and trusted relationships with pediatric providers and worry about moving into the adult care environment, which was viewed as more clinical and less caring. This was expressed in a variety of ways, including a feeling of "culture shock" with individuals having to learn new ways to communicate with their healthcare teams. In AYA with chronic conditions that are life-shortening, such as cystic fibrosis or congenital heart disease, additional themes emerge around transition, including social isolation, physical incapacity, treatment burden, and the potential need to make different choices for career and family compared to healthy peers [10, 14].

The anxiety regarding transition is often heightened in parents who worry about their child as he or she learns to navigate the adult healthcare system more independently. Often parental anxiety is perceived by HCP as greater than that of the transitioning AYA. Moreover, within adult care, the parent often becomes relegated to the sidelines after being the primary point of contact throughout a child's life prior to transition. Parents may not trust their AYA to take on the roles and responsibilities of an adult and worry that they would not receive health-related information to assist their child in navigating the adult healthcare system. Parents also have trusted relationships with pediatric care providers that they will be leaving behind. In adult care, the parent is not likely to develop the same level of trust given the shift in focus of care and the growing independence of the AYA. Parents are also more likely to worry about the quality of care received in the adult health system.

Provider Experience of Transition

For HCPs, the qualitative research on transition sometimes differs between pediatric and adult care providers. Pediatric providers are much more likely to believe that transfer of care should not be based upon age alone, but rather milestones of development. In contrast, adult HCPs often feel that a policy regarding the age of transition helps create a more well-defined set of expectations around transition [8, 12]. Both pediatric and adult providers note that parents are more resistant to transition than the young adult (YA) [8, 12]. Adult HCPs note that the transition into the adult healthcare system is difficult at times because AYA are perceived as being "overprotected" in the pediatric environment and may not be fully aware of their health condition [15]. Both pediatric and adult HCPs agree there are a variety of paths for transition and sometimes the lack of availability of adult HCPs limits the ability to transition [16]. In addition, the perceived differences in the healthcare environment can also be a barrier to transition, with the adult environment perceived as more business-like and less holistic [17].

Using Qualitative Outcomes to Guide Transition Programs

Given the themes noted in qualitative studies of transition, multiple recommendations can be made to guide development of transition programs and future research. As the AYA plans for transition, there are many challenges faced by the AYA and their caregivers. An initial recommendation based upon qualitative findings is that programs should develop written transition practices and policies that are shared with AYA and their caregivers. This is the first key tenet of the Got Transition program, a transition readiness program developed by the National Alliance to Advance Adolescent Health (https://www.gottransition.org/six-core-elements/). In addition, AYA should be evaluated for transition readiness at regular intervals, and transfer plans can be individualized with input from AYA and caregivers. A common finding of the qualitative research was that age should not be the primary arbiter of transfer of care, but rather should be one of the many factors considered when an individual transfers to adult care. In AYA who are struggling with self-management skills, additional time for education and support may be required prior to transfer. The AYA may benefit from more one-on-one guidance from a member of the pediatric team, such as a nurse with specific training on transition readiness. Future qualitative studies may be focused on how AYA, caregivers, and HCPs experience programs that have been developed for transition. Other areas for qualitative research include quality improvement within the transition program, better understanding of how transition programs can prepare AYA for adult life outside of the healthcare transition (school, career choices, relationships), and assessing the needs of the AYA regarding inpatient care as a facet of transition. In addition, the qualitative assessment and development of group transition programs for AYA with chronic illnesses could be explored. Another avenue for future research is to employ mixed-methods research combining qualitative and quantitative research. One example of this would be determining how an AYA perceives transition and how this impacts specific health outcomes after transition.

Overview of Quantitative Research in Transition Medicine

Quantitative research forms the basis of most research that is performed in medicine. It involves the systematic collection of variables that can be quantified for determination of the effect on specific outcomes utilizing statistical analysis. Quantitative research can be performed in many ways, including observation or measurement of the effects of an intervention. Data can be collected prospectively or retrospectively. Individuals or groups of individuals can be randomized to receive an intervention and may or may not be blinded to the intervention that is occurring. In the realm of transition medicine, some specific tools have been developed to measure transition readiness. In addition, transition programs, usually at a single center, have been studied to assess the effects of these programs on outcomes. Common outcome measures for quantitative transition research can include a variety of clinical measures that can be general (patient and parent satisfaction, hospitalizations, successful transfer, or care) or disease-specific (hemoglobin A1C in type 1 diabetes mellitus, graft failure in kidney transplantation, or lung function in cystic fibrosis). In this section, we will review these tools that have been developed and some of the measurable outcomes that can be used to assess transition success.

Tools for Measuring Transition Readiness

Measuring and tracking transition readiness is one of the core principles outlined by the National Alliance to Advance Adolescent Health in the Got Transition program [18]. Transition readiness can be defined as indicators that an AYA and his or her caregivers are prepared to complete the process of transfer into adult care. Transition readiness should be measurable with components that are modifiable with intervention or education and can be tracked over time [19]. Multiple transition readiness assessments have been developed, and some have been modified for disease-specific assessment of transition readiness. However, most available tools, including the transition readiness assessment available at Got Transition, have not been externally validated [18]. In a systematic review evaluating the psychometric properties of transition readiness questionnaires, ten instruments were included in the analysis; however, many of these reported limited validity and reliability data, often based on one study [19]. Some questionnaires have been validated as disease-specific measures in cystic fibrosis, kidney transplant, liver transplant, sickle cell disease, and HIV [19]. Among the generic transition readiness assessments, the Transition Readiness Assessment Questionnaire (TRAQ) [20, 21] and the Self-Management and Transition to Adulthood with Rx = Treatment Questionnaire (STARx)) [22, 23] are the most frequently used patient-administered instruments. The TRxANSITION Index is an alternative instrument administered by a trained member of the healthcare team. When the commonly used instruments are compared, the TRAQ focuses on individual behaviors without assessment in disease knowledge, whereas the STARx and the TRxANSITION Index both include a combination of behaviors and disease knowledge [24]. Criticisms of current transition readiness assessments have included the use of convenience samples for testing and validation, lack of diverse subjects, lack of inclusion of stakeholders, and inadequate data regarding how the instruments can be utilized to target transition interventions [19].

Transition Readiness Assessment Questionnaire (TRAQ)

The TRAQ was developed to measure healthcare behaviors and self-management skills that help an AYA successfully transition to adult health care [20, 21]. Its development was based upon the stages of change model with two primary domains identified through initial factor analysis—Skills for Self-Management and Skills for Self-Advocacy [20, 21, 25]. The self-administered questionnaire asks 20 items across five areas, including managing medications, appointment keeping, tracking health issues, talking with providers, and managing daily activities such as meals and cleaning [21]. An AYA can respond in one of five answers as outlined in Table 2.1, with a score between 1 and 5 on each item. Total score and domain scores are determined by the average overall score and average score within each domain.

Table 2.1 TRAQ responses as related to the stages of change model

TRAQ response	TRAQ score	Stage	Definition
No, I do not know how	1	Pre-contemplation	No planned change over next 6 months
No, but I want to learn	2	Contemplation	Aware a problem exists and intends to take action, usually within 6 months
No, but I am learning	3	Preparation	Intends to take action within the next 30 days and report some behavioral steps
Yes, I have started doing this	4	Action	Has changed behavior within last 6 months
Yes, I always do this	5	Maintenance	Has changed behavior for more than 6 months

Adapted from Sawicki et al. [20]

In a chronic disease population, older age was shown to be associated with higher scores, but other variables including insurance status and gender did not [21]. The instrument may be given repeatedly every 6–12 months to assess changes in TRAQ scores over time. No published data has demonstrated whether longitudinal changes in TRAQ scores are associated with outcomes specific to transition, such as successful transfer of care or satisfaction with transition.

Self-Management and Transition to Adulthood with Rx = Treatment Questionnaire (STARx)

The STARx questionnaire was developed with input from AYA, their caregivers, and multidisciplinary providers in the United States, England, and Mexico. Over 1000 AYA with chronic illness from the ages of 8–25 participated in the development of the STARx questionnaire over its phases of development. The self-administered questionnaire has 18 questions scored on a Likert scale from 0 to 5 over three domains with a total score between 0 and 90 with higher scores indicating more knowledge of skills deemed important for healthcare transition [22, 23]. The three domains assessed include communication with medical providers, disease knowledge, and self-management. In validation testing, STARx scores correlated positively with TRAQ scores and higher STARx scores were associated with greater medication adherence, but not healthcare utilization [22]. A parental questionnaire has also been developed to assess the parent's view of AYA readiness for transition. Overall, parents score a child's transition readiness significantly lower than the AYA although there is a moderately strong correlation between child and parent scores ($r = 0.58$). The domain with the greatest positive correlation was disease knowledge, while an AYA and parent were most likely to differ in the area of self-management [26].

The TRxANSITION Index

The TRxANSITION Index is a 32-item questionnaire that is administered by a trained member of the healthcare team. It evaluates transition readiness across ten domains: type of chronic health condition, Rx/medications, adherence, nutrition, self-management skills, issues of reproduction, trade/school, insurance, ongoing support, and new healthcare providers. Each item is scored as 0, 0.5, or 1.0 based upon skill acquisition with a total score between 0 and 10 with higher scores indicating more skills pertinent to transition [27]. This instrument has been given to a large cohort of individuals ($n = 566$) over a period of 10 years who completed the survey at least twice, and 232 individuals had more than 2 scores [28]. Factors associated with increases in TRxANSITION Index included older age and female gender. However, as individuals age, there are smaller gains in the TRxANSITION Index over time. Lower scores were associated with intellectual limitations, living farther from the tertiary care center, and having no insurance [28]. Age was also associated with skill achievement on subscales of the instrument. When skill achievement is defined as the age at which the average subscale score first passed 75% proficiency, individuals in the youngest category (age 12–14) had early mastery of adherence and ongoing support, but it was not until older ages when issues of reproduction (ages 19–20) and self-management skills and insurance (age > 20) were achieved [28].

Evaluation of Transition Interventions or Comprehensive Transition Programs

Comprehensive transition programs, such as Got Transition, have been developed at the national level, and locally in healthcare institutions, a variety of interventions have been implemented to support AYA transitioning to adult care. A large systematic review published in 2017 identified 43 studies looking at outcomes of structured pediatric to adult healthcare transition interventions [29]. Slightly more than half were considered moderate to strong in overall quality. Selection bias was a prominent issue across included studies as all but five interventions were targeted to a single medical condition and most had small sample sizes. Moreover, no studies evaluated the experiences of healthy adolescents [29]. The positive outcomes associated with structured transition interventions were divided into the following categories: population health (adherence, quality of life, self-care), experience of care (patient satisfaction, barriers to care), and utilization and cost outcomes. Sixty-five percent of included studies reported a significant positive outcome [29]. Interventions studied varied from transition preparation, often with a focus on self-management and disease education, to transfer of care activities including transition clinics or explicit transfer of care plans. A different review noted that testing of healthcare transition models remains in an early state of development, particularly with regard to design and implementation of high-quality studies, and advocated for funding of large multisite studies [30]. Thus, given the limited data available, it is hard to know which components of transition programs are the most beneficial in improving outcomes.

Transition Outcome Measures

As comprehensive transition programs are implemented, it is imperative to have outcome measures to evaluate the interventions. In prior studies, a variety of outcome measures have been used and can be framed within the quadruple aim framework as identified previously in Fig. 2.1: health outcomes, patient experience, provider experience, and cost of care.

Health Outcomes

Health outcomes cover a wide range of measures from specific factors around a disease state to quality of life and self-efficacy. While the health outcomes that have been assessed in transition research can be more generalized, disease-specific outcomes are more commonly utilized. The largest number of studies of transition interventions has been performed in AYA with type 1 diabetes mellitus (T1DM). A variety of outcome measures have been assessed for T1DM, including hemoglobin A1C, weight, microalbuminuria, and standard eye and foot examinations [29], with transition interventions showing an improvement in these measures. In other diseases, the outcomes would be chosen to reflect the clinically important measures for maintaining disease control. For kidney or liver transplant, levels of immunosuppression have been used [29]. In lung diseases, the outcome measure may be lung function in cystic fibrosis [31, 32] or measures of asthma control in youth with asthma. For many childhood diseases, transition programs have not been studied well. Thus, the best outcome measures are yet to be defined. More generically, adherence to prescribed treatments after transition can be assessed by medication-possession ratios and/or self-report [22, 33].

Patient-reported quality of life (QOL) is a health outcome measure that can be affected by transition interventions [29]. A variety of QOL measures have been developed and can be generic or disease specific. To assess the effects of a transition program, QOL has been measured as an outcome in many diseases. In general, transition programs have improved well-being as measured by global well-being scores or disease activity scores [29]. As noted in the section above, many transition readiness scales measure engagement in care and self-management. A study in 80 individuals with T1DM demonstrated that a nurse-led transition education improved disease knowledge and ability to self-adjust insulin doses [34]. This intensive program included group sessions and required an estimated 12–15 hours per patient over a 6-month period. Thus, the time intensity of the program may be difficult for other centers to replicate, and whether the improvement could have been realized by patients beyond transition age was not explored. In juvenile rheumatoid arthritis, a multisite study in the United Kingdom that enrolled 359 patients and families in a structured transition program showed improvement in both QOL and measures of disease knowledge when assessed over 12 months [35].

Finally, assessing the value of transition programs in preventing excess morbidity or mortality is a possible outcome for transition interventions. In general, small sample sizes, single center nature of studies, and short follow-up prevent transition programs from determining this effect. One study in AYA with renal transplants showed that having a transition coordinator improved graft function and delayed time to death [36]. Another study of a transition program in renal transplant at a different institution also showed similar findings of decreased graft loss or death using historical controls as a comparator [37]. Both studies were small with ≤20 individuals in the intervention groups, and the comparison group in each was a historical control [36, 37]. Thus, care should be taken in interpretation of these results given advances in medical care over time that could explain differences in outcomes.

Patient Experience

A second goal of the quadruple aim is to improve patient experience through structured transition programs. Some studies have evaluated internally developed surveys, specifically given for the purpose of assessing their programs, and have shown improved patient satisfaction regarding transition preparation and transfer of care [38–41]. A specific instrument called "Mind the Gap" has been developed for assessing patient satisfaction with transitional care in the pediatric environment prior to transfer [42]. The instrument was originally developed for use in patients with juvenile rheumatoid arthritis but has since been adapted for use in other disease states. This instrument has versions for both the parent (27 items) and adolescent (22 items) and asks questions across three domains: environment, provider characteristics, and process issues. Individuals are asked to rate their perception of current care on a 1–7 Likert scale and also to rate what his or her expectations of "best care" would be. The "gap" is the difference between current and best care on each item [42]. A score of 0 reflects no gap (i.e., no difference between current care and best care), whereas a positive score would indicate that current care is not rated as highly as perceived best care, hence the gap. Negative scores are possible and would indicate that current care exceeds what is expected of best care [42]. Examples of questions in each domain are included in Table 2.2. In the initial survey development in juvenile rheumatoid arthritis, parents reported larger gaps compared to their AYA, particularly in the domains of environment and process issues, although median gaps for all domains were 1 point or less [42]. In a study in the United Kingdom, the

Table 2.2 Sample question from "Mind the Gap" transition satisfaction survey

Domain	Sample questions
Managing the environment	Has a physical environment that caters for my (son/daughter's) age group (e.g., appropriate decoration, teenage magazines)
	Does not waste my (son/daughter's) time at the clinic
	Provides appointments that are convenient for me (and my son/daughter)
	Provides opportunities to meet other parents of young people with *disease state* (parent only)
Provider characteristics	Allow me (my son/daughter) to decide who should be in the examination room
	Has staff who are very knowledgeable about *disease state* and the latest treatment
	Has staff who know me (my son/daughter) well
	Provides me with honest explanations of my son/daughter's condition and treatment options, including side effects (parent only)
Process issues	Has a named member of the staff who is responsible for coordinating my (son/daughter's) care
	Helps me (and my son/daughter) plan for my/their future
	Helps me (and my son/daughter) prepare for my move to adult services
	Helps me support my son/daughter's independence (parent only)

Adapted from Shaw et al. [42]

Mind the Gap survey was given at 4 time points to a cohort of 374 individuals with one of three diagnoses (autism spectrum disorder, cerebral palsy, or T1DM) [43]. Over the time period of interest, 54% of individuals transferred into adult services and an additional 28% transferred into primary care. It was also noted that the parent's satisfaction (the gap) was worse than that of the AYA [43]. At baseline, the gap between the differing diagnoses was similar but did worsen at subsequent visits for both cerebral palsy and autism spectrum disorders [43]. Perhaps this reflects an adult healthcare system that is more available and prepared to accept some chronic diseases (T1DM) over more complex childhood diseases (cerebral palsy, autism spectrum disorder).

Healthcare Utilization

The third aspect of the quadruple aim is to understand how transition programs affect healthcare utilization and costs to the healthcare system. Less data is available to assess this aim. Large-scale transition programs can be costly requiring the dedication of a team member, typically a nurse, to administer the program. The direct benefits to the health system can be difficult to ascertain. When costs are considered, very few publications have reported on this outcome. In T1DM, individuals in a young adult clinic for those between ages 15 and 25 had fewer admissions for diabetic ketoacidosis than those not served by these services. This difference led to an estimated hospital savings of $130,500 yearly after accounting for the salary of the nurse educator [44]. In one study of renal transplant patients, there was no difference in yearly cost per patient in those who had undergone the transition program vs. the cost estimates of historical controls [37]. However, the authors asserted that the transition program led to less graft loss; thus it was cost-effective as the cost per patient would be lower than the cost of sustaining someone on dialysis [37]. In a study in the United Kingdom, transfer of care to adult services resulted in an overall drop in yearly median expense to the healthcare system by £302, although this was not statistically significant [43]. In this analysis, potentially beneficial factors associated with transition were assessed for cost-effectiveness. While some features were felt to be potentially beneficial, the conclusion of this analysis was that these services were unlikely to reduce costs to the National Health Service and could actually increase them [43]. Other studies have shown that participation in a transition program led to fewer hospitalizations and greater engagement with adult healthcare services. In one study of 72 AYA with inflammatory bowel disease, the individuals who participated in the transition program had fewer hospitalizations and emergency surgeries [45]. A historical control was utilized; thus, differences in care or practice of health care during this time is a confounding variable. In order to attempt to control for time of follow-up, hospitalizations and surgeries were limited to the 2 years after transition in both groups [45]. In T1DM, a young adult clinic for individuals aged 15–25 utilized a diabetes educator as a transition coordinator and enrolled 191 individuals in the program [46]. Over the period of the program, hospital admissions for diabetic ketoacidosis decreased by 33%, and for those hospitalized, the length of stay decreased by 1.1 days [46]. Regarding engagement in care, individuals who participated in a transition program had higher rates of attendance at adult care appointments [40, 45–48]. In addition, studies have demonstrated that a structured transition program led to a decrease time to the first appointment in adult care and fewer lapses in care [49–51].

Provider Experience

Provider experience has been added to the quality improvement framework to become the fourth aim in the quadruple aim [4]. At this time, there is no specific data available regarding provider experiences with transition programs. In the era of increasing time demands on physicians and team members, assessing the impact of implementing transition programs will be important for the future of these programs. It is well-known that physician and nursing burnout is an increasing problem in health care. Implementing the six core elements of transition could add extra time to a clinical visit as well as additional documentation. In the development of programs, care should be taken to include all team members and patient-family partners to co-produce a transition program that will be both beneficial and efficient. Developing these programs will also require resources and support from the healthcare system to ensure that the burden of implementation does not fall onto individuals who may be overburdened. Future research should be performed to assess the experience of transition programs from the provider standpoint as well.

Future Research Agenda

With an ever-expanding population of AYA with chronic illnesses of childhood ageing into the adult healthcare system, transition from pediatric to adult healthcare services is a growing field. As the six core elements of transition are implemented more broadly and in a greater number of clinics, many questions remain unanswered. Most studies are single-centered and often study only a single disease state. To generate a more comprehensive body of transition research, a recent statement published by the American Academy of Pediatrics, the American Academy of Family Physicians, and the American College of Physicians outlined key factors that should be addressed in future research into transition. These include incorporating all three components (transition preparation, transfer, and integration into adult care) of transition into study design and evaluating both processes and outcomes [52]. Future outcomes from transition research should be couched in the quadruple aim framework, including population health outcomes, patient experience, and utilization and cost savings [52], but also including provider experience. Long-term outcomes of transition programs have also not been evaluated. National health surveys are encouraged to also help frame transition research. The Cochrane Collaboration also highlighted areas for transition research focusing on study design and methods that can lead to better knowledge around transition practices, particularly which elements of an intervention contribute to its effectiveness [53]. Multicenter and innovative study designs, including pragmatic trials, should be considered in future study design. In addition, future research needs to be more transparent about inclusivity to ensure that a wide range of ethnicities and socioeconomic backgrounds are recruited into studies of healthcare transition.

Conclusion

Transition research encompasses a wide body of potential study designs and outcomes. At present, much remains to be done to fully understand best transition practices and their impacts on outcomes on AYA, both with and without chronic illness. Qualitative studies can inform development of transition programs and lead to future quantitative outcome measures. Developing tools that are validated and reliable to measure factors within transition such as transition readiness and transition satisfaction helps researchers as they plan future trials. Framing outcomes in the quadruple aim framework is beneficial to understand the current state of the literature and inform future research.

References

1. Surgeon general's conference: growing up and getting medical care: youth with special health care needs: a summary of conference proceedings. U.S Public Health Service; 1989.
2. Children with special health care needs: NSCH data brief; 2020.
3. Lebrun-Harris LA, et al. Transition planning among US youth with and without special health care needs. Pediatrics. 2018;142(4):e20180194.
4. Bodenheimer T, Sinsky C. From triple to quadruple aim: care of the patient requires care of the provider. Ann Fam Med. 2014;12(6):573–6.
5. Pope C, van Royen P, Baker R. Qualitative methods in research on healthcare quality. Qual Saf Health Care. 2002;11(2):148–52.
6. Padgett DK. Qualitative and mixed methods in public health. Thousand Oaks: SAGE Publications, Inc; 2012.
7. Broad KL, et al. Youth experiences of transition from child mental health services to adult mental health services: a qualitative thematic synthesis. BMC Psychiatry. 2017;17(1):380.
8. Coyne I, et al. Healthcare transition for adolescents and young adults with long-term conditions: qualitative study of patients, parents and healthcare professionals' experiences. J Clin Nurs. 2019;28(21–22):4062–76.
9. Fegran L, et al. Adolescents' and young adults' transition experiences when transferring from paediatric to adult care: a qualitative metasynthesis. Int J Nurs Stud. 2014;51(1):123–35.
10. Jamieson N, et al. Children's experiences of cystic fibrosis: a systematic review of qualitative studies. Pediatrics. 2014;133(6):e1683.
11. Tuchman LK, Slap GB, Britto MT. Transition to adult care: experiences and expectations of adolescents with a chronic illness. Child Care Health Dev. 2008;34(5):557–63.
12. van Staa AL, et al. Crossing the transition chasm: experiences and recommendations for improving transitional care of young adults, parents and providers. Child Care Health Dev. 2011;37(6):821–32.
13. Tong A, et al. Adolescent views on transition in diabetes and nephrology. Eur J Pediatr. 2013;172(3):293–304.
14. Chong LSH, et al. Children's experiences of congenital heart disease: a systematic review of qualitative studies. Eur J Pediatr. 2018;177(3):319–36.
15. McLoughlin A, Matthews C, Hickey TM. "They're kept in a bubble": healthcare professionals' views on transitioning young adults with congenital heart disease from paediatric to adult care. Child Care Health Dev. 2018;44(5):736–45.
16. Cruikshank M, et al. Transitional care in clinical networks for young people with juvenile idiopathic arthritis: current situation and challenges. Clin Rheumatol. 2016;35(4):893–9.
17. Burke L, et al. The transition of adolescents with juvenile idiopathic arthritis or epilepsy from paediatric health-care services to adult health-care services: a scoping review of the literature and a synthesis of the evidence. J Child Health Care. 2018;22(3):332–58.
18. White PH, et al. Six core elements of transition 3.0: an implementation guide. In: Got transition. Washington, DC: The National Alliance to Advance Adolescent Health; 2020.
19. Schwartz LA, et al. Measures of readiness to transition to adult health care for youth with chronic physical health conditions: a systematic review and recommendations for measurement testing and development. J Pediatr Psychol. 2014;39(6):588–601.
20. Sawicki GS, et al. Measuring the transition readiness of youth with special healthcare needs: validation of the TRAQ--Transition Readiness Assessment Questionnaire. J Pediatr Psychol. 2011;36(2):160–71.
21. Wood DL, et al. The Transition Readiness Assessment Questionnaire (TRAQ): its factor structure, reliability, and validity. Acad Pediatr. 2014;14(4):415–22.
22. Cohen SE, et al. Self-management and transition readiness assessment: concurrent, predictive and discriminant validation of the STARx questionnaire. J Pediatr Nurs. 2015;30(5):668–76.
23. Ferris M, et al. Self-management and transition readiness assessment: development, reliability, and factor structure of the STARx questionnaire. J Pediatr Nurs. 2015;30(5):691–9.

24. Straus EJ. Challenges in measuring healthcare transition readiness: taking stock and looking forward. J Pediatr Nurs. 2019;46:109–17.
25. Prochaska JO, DiClemente CC, Norcross JC. In search of how people change: applications to addictive behaviors. Am Psychol. 1992;47(9):1102–14.
26. Nazareth M, et al. A parental report of youth transition readiness: the parent STARx questionnaire (STARx-P) and re-evaluation of the STARx child report. J Pediatr Nurs. 2018;38:122–6.
27. Ferris ME, et al. A clinical tool to measure the components of health-care transition from pediatric care to adult care: the UNC TR(x)ANSITION scale. Ren Fail. 2012;34(6):744–53.
28. Zhong Y, et al. Longitudinal self-management and/or transition readiness per the TRxANSITION index among patients with chronic conditions in pediatric or adult care settings. J Pediatr. 2018;203:361–370.e1.
29. Gabriel P, et al. Outcome evidence for structured pediatric to adult health care transition interventions: a systematic review. J Pediatr. 2017;188:263–269.e15.
30. Betz CL, et al. Systematic review: health care transition practice service models. Nurs Outlook. 2016;64(3):229–43.
31. Duguépéroux I, et al. Clinical changes of patients with cystic fibrosis during transition from pediatric to adult care. J Adolesc Health. 2008;43(5):459–65.
32. Tuchman L, Schwartz M. Health outcomes associated with transition from pediatric to adult cystic fibrosis care. Pediatrics. 2013;132(5):847–53.
33. McQuillan RF, et al. Benefits of a transfer clinic in adolescent and young adult kidney transplant patients. Can J Kidney Health Dis. 2015;2:45.
34. Vidal M, et al. Impact of a special therapeutic education programme in patients transferred from a paediatric to an adult diabetes unit. Eur Diabetes Nurs. 2004;1(1):23–7.
35. McDonagh JE, et al. The impact of a coordinated transitional care programme on adolescents with juvenile idiopathic arthritis. Rheumatology. 2007;46(1):161–8.
36. Annunziato RA, et al. Strangers headed to a strange land? A pilot study of using a transition coordinator to improve transfer from pediatric to adult services. J Pediatr. 2013;163(6):1628–33.
37. Prestidge C, et al. Utility and cost of a renal transplant transition clinic. Pediatr Nephrol. 2012;27(2):295–302.
38. Chaudhry SR, Keaton M, Nasr SZ. Evaluation of a cystic fibrosis transition program from pediatric to adult care. Pediatr Pulmonol. 2013;48(7):658–65.
39. Pape L, et al. Different models of transition to adult care after pediatric kidney transplantation: a comparative study. Pediatr Transplant. 2013;17(6):518–24.
40. Cadario F, et al. Transition process of patients with type 1 diabetes (T1DM) from paediatric to the adult health care service: a hospital-based approach. Clin Endocrinol (Oxf). 2009;71(3):346–50.
41. Jurasek L, Ray L, Quigley D. Development and implementation of an adolescent epilepsy transition clinic. J Neurosci Nurs. 2010;42(4):181–9.
42. Shaw KL, et al. Development and preliminary validation of the 'Mind the Gap' scale to assess satisfaction with transitional health care among adolescents with juvenile idiopathic arthritis. Child Care Health Dev. 2007;33(4):380–8.
43. Colver A, et al. Facilitating the transition of young people with long-term conditions through health services from childhood to adulthood: the transition research programme. Programme Grants Appl Res. 2019;7(4):1–244.
44. Burns K, et al. Access to a youth-specific service for young adults with type 1 diabetes mellitus is associated with decreased hospital length of stay for diabetic ketoacidosis. Intern Med J. 2018;48(4):396–402.
45. Cole R, et al. Evaluation of outcomes in adolescent inflammatory bowel disease patients following transfer from pediatric to adult health care services: case for transition. J Adolesc Health. 2015;57(2):212–7.
46. Holmes-Walker DJ, Llewellyn AC, Farrell K. A transition care programme which improves diabetes control and reduces hospital admission rates in young adults with type 1 diabetes aged 15–25 years. Diabet Med. 2007;24(7):764–9.

47. Hankins JS, et al. A transition pilot program for adolescents with sickle cell disease. J Pediatr Health Care. 2012;26(6):e45–9.
48. Fredericks EM, et al. Quality improvement targeting adherence during the transition from a pediatric to adult liver transplant clinic. J Clin Psychol Med Settings. 2015;22(2):150–9.
49. Hergenroeder AC, et al. Functional classification of heart failure before and after implementing a healthcare transition program for youth and young adults transferring from a pediatric to an adult congenital heart disease clinics. Congenit Heart Dis. 2018;13(4):548–53.
50. Jones MR, et al. Transfer from pediatric to adult endocrinology. Endocr Pract. 2017;23(7):822–30.
51. Mackie AS, et al. Transition intervention for adolescents with congenital heart disease. J Am Coll Cardiol. 2018;71(16):1768–77.
52. White PH, Cooley WC. Supporting the health care transition from adolescence to adulthood in the medical home. Pediatrics. 2018;142(5):e20182587.
53. Campbell F, et al. Transition of care for adolescents from paediatric services to adult health services. Cochrane Database Syst Rev. 2016;(4):CD009794.

Chapter 3
Training Trainees: Creating a Better Workforce to Support Transition Care

Rachel Quaney and Stephen Kirkby

Importance of Teaching Healthcare Transition

Advances in recent decades have allowed children with chronic disorders to survive much longer than previously, often reaching adulthood. Patients with traditional pediatric diseases, who in prior years may have remained under the care of pediatric teams until end of life, now need to transition care to adult providers. Increasing recognition of the importance of the healthcare transition process, as well as the pitfalls, has led various medical organizations to issue formal recommendations. Most notably, a clinical report issued by the American Academy of Pediatrics (AAP), American Academy of Family Physicians (AAFP), and American College of Physicians (ACP) has undergone multiple iterations in its quest to delineate the need for healthcare transition programs and the recommended processes [1–3].

Despite several decades of attention being paid to this process of transition, progress has been slow, and implementation has remained low. Reasons cited for low rates of transitional programs are varied, including lack of comfort with or training in congenital and childhood disorders, lack of time or reimbursement, uncertainty regarding roles and responsibilities, difficulty navigating systems issues and

R. Quaney (✉)
Division of Pulmonary, Critical Care & Sleep Medicine, Department of Internal Medicine, The Ohio State University Wexner Medical Center, Columbus, OH, USA
e-mail: rachel.quaney@osumc.edu

S. Kirkby
Division of Pulmonary, Critical Care & Sleep Medicine, Department of Internal Medicine, The Ohio State University Wexner Medical Center, Columbus, OH, USA

Section of Pulmonary Medicine, Nationwide Children's Hospital, Columbus, OH, USA
e-mail: Stephen.Kirkby@nationwidechildrens.org

© Springer Nature Switzerland AG 2021
C. D. Brown, E. Crowley (eds.), *Transitioning Care from Pediatric to Adult Pulmonology*, Respiratory Medicine,
https://doi.org/10.1007/978-3-030-68688-8_3

transition coordination, addressing psychosocial needs and patient maturation, and mediating family involvement [4–6]. Despite transition guidelines being available almost two decades ago, these issues continue to be mentioned by practicing physicians [1, 7]. Based on how long transition guidelines have existed, one would think that training programs would have well-established transition curriculums and therefore newer graduates would be better equipped to tackle these challenges. However, the review of medical education does not corroborate this assumption. In fact, very few residents and fellows report confidence in performing transition care, and a majority report no education about the transition process [8, 9].

Importance of Teaching Healthcare Transition Specific to Pulmonology

Like many other fields, pulmonology must also prepare for healthcare transition, but the implementation of programs and education has not kept pace with the need. The adoption of comprehensive transition protocols remains inadequate, even in areas such as cystic fibrosis, which has been leading the field of pulmonology in terms of healthcare transition [7]. It follows that care transition programs and protocols are even less established for other pulmonary disorders. Of accredited pediatric pulmonary programs in the United States, 78.1% do not use a standardized transition process, and 41.4% have no transition process at all [10]. This is not for lack of need, as there are currently 24.8 million children aged 12–17 years requiring transition care in the United States, and over 6 million of these children have special health care needs, many with pulmonary disorders or respiratory technology dependence [11]. Meanwhile, there are less than 1200 pediatric pulmonologists and 15,000 adult physicians currently certified in pulmonary or pulmonary and critical care medicine [12, 13].

This shortage of pediatric pulmonologists and the projected shortage of adult pulmonologists in the coming years is due to a combination of an aging workforce but also aging pediatric patients preparing to "graduate" to adult medical care, since 90% of children with chronic conditions now survive into adulthood [14]. This current cohort of physicians cannot meet the needs of our adolescent and young adult pulmonary patients preparing for healthcare transition unless a concerted effort is made focusing on improved training. Because, if we continue to build transition clinics and transition protocols without adequately addressing the pipeline of health professionals, who will be responsible for the implementation and utilization of these resources? Therefore, there is an urgent need to develop a transition curriculum for our pulmonary training programs, so we can focus on the current fellows who will soon be emerging as a critical portion of this workforce.

While the AAP, AAFP, and ACP recognize this importance of preparing physicians in transition care, the goals set forth are for all physicians providing care for children and young adults with special medical needs. There is no separate set of goals for trainees or for training program leadership. The AAP, AAFP, and ACP recommend physicians to (1) understand the rationale for transition from child-oriented to adult-oriented health care, (2) have the knowledge and skills to facilitate transition, and (3) know if, how, and when transfer of care is indicated [1, 2]. In order for practicing physicians to achieve these goals, healthcare transition education should begin in medical school and continue throughout post-graduate training and beyond [5, 6].

Education in congenital and childhood-onset conditions has been shown to be a critical factor in the comfort of internists accepting care of young adults with special medical needs [6]. Furthermore, adult physicians who were exposed to the process of transitioning health care during residency training were more likely to feel comfortable accepting new young adults as patients [5]. Despite this, the Accreditation Council for Graduate Medical Education (ACGME) Next Accreditation System common program requirements for residency programs and fellowship programs do not address the transition process of young adults [15, 16]. However, the updated ACGME Program Requirements for Graduate Medical Education in Pediatric Pulmonology has recently incorporated this initiative, adding that "fellows must be able to facilitate the transition of patients with pulmonary disorders from pediatrics to adult health care settings" [17]. No similar updates have been made to the Program Requirements for Adult Pulmonary Disease or Pulmonary Disease and Critical Care Medicine [18, 19].

Adult pulmonary training programs are not required to provide their trainees with opportunities for pediatric exposure, despite other specialties offering a framework. For example, the training for sleep medicine, anesthesiology, radiology, and otorhinolaryngology requires pediatric rotations, and various surgical fields have pediatric rotations available, although these are variable depending on the training program. Within the primary care realm, family medicine and combined internal medicine-pediatrics (IM-Peds) programs are ideally suited for models of transition care training, but in fact IM-Peds is the only residency specialty that explicitly includes transition education in their ACGME program requirements [20, 21]. In spite of the available examples for how to incorporate transition education into training, adult pulmonary training program requirements are not alone in their oversight. Many specialties and subspecialties have common program requirements and milestones that allude to "transitions" that in fact are referring to handoffs between phases of care, such as inpatient to outpatient or vice versa [18, 19]. While some IM-Peds graduates do pursue pulmonary fellowship, this small number of individuals cannot fill the current void of physicians needed for pulmonary healthcare transition.

If our internal medicine and pediatric residents do not graduate feeling capable of executing healthcare transition, and our pulmonary fellowship training programs do not have a designated curriculum to address this need, we will continue to produce pulmonologists largely unprepared to care for this population. In fact, the field of pulmonology currently has no existing guidelines or even literature about transition training. This marked disparity between the future need for pulmonologists trained in transition care and the current shortage of associated curriculum needs to be addressed.

Key Topics for a Transition Curriculum in Pulmonology

Curriculum development for healthcare transition should be multifaceted and build upon what has already been done in other specialties. A survey of medical professionals with expertise in healthcare transition identified five goals to guide designing transition curriculum for primary care residents [22]. These goals include the following: (1) understand transition from pediatric to adult health care, (2) understand key insurance and social service issues, (3) consider developmental and psychosocial issues, (4) address educational/vocational needs, and (5) improve healthcare systems [22]. However, these are not all encompassing and likely run the risk of leaving out key elements. A transition curriculum for pulmonary trainees should include both the medical knowledge about congenital and childhood disease entities and particulars about the transition process.

Disease Entities

In order to ensure adult providers welcoming young adults into their practice have the knowledge and expertise required, educational efforts must be made to address both diseases unique to childhood as well as the ones seen across the lifespan. Diseases that need to be addressed include cystic fibrosis, asthma, bronchopulmonary dysplasia, interstitial lung disease, lung transplantation, sleep disorders, neuromuscular disorders, and chronic respiratory insufficiency such as respiratory technology dependence (i.e., chronic ventilator use).

In addition to covering pathology, adult pulmonary training regarding transition care should also attend to variations in physiology. Pediatric care focuses on growth and development of their patients, whereas adult medicine attends primarily to senescence. This is a key variation in practice, as young adults are still growing and developing, even as they enter the world of adult medicine. For example, the continued growth of a young adult has implications for things such as the interpretation of pulmonary function tests.

While these topics of pathophysiology are addressed in pediatric pulmonary training programs, they will need to be added to or expanded upon in adult pulmonary training programs. The importance of educating about these diseases is evidenced by how often medical knowledge is cited as a barrier for healthcare transition implementation [5, 6, 23].

Process of Transition

However, knowing about these disease entities is not enough, because healthcare transitions are much more than medical knowledge. The process of transition must also be addressed. It is important to note the transition process includes actual transfer of care from pediatric to adult physicians, but transition is much more comprehensive and also more nuanced.

Transition encompasses the process of preparing and building skills to become an active participant in adult care, whereas transfer is the discrete time point when a patient is first seen in adult care. The National Center for Health Care Transition lays out Six Core Elements of Health Care Transition™, defined as (1) transition policy, (2) transition tracking and monitoring, (3) transition readiness, (4) transition planning, (5) transfer of care, and (6) transfer completion and ongoing care [24]. It will be imperative to teach both pediatric and adult trainees about the complete transition process, as well as how to incorporate these elements into their current and future practice. Pediatric pulmonologists should be competent in elements one through five and familiar with what ongoing adult care constitutes in order to best care for these patients and receive feedback on their processes. On the other hand, adult pulmonologists should be competent in all elements of transfer but still be familiar with earlier stages of transition and be able to participate in transition planning if their practice environment allows or requires their input.

Psychosocial Transition

How a patient with one of these pulmonary diseases progresses through the Six Core Elements of Health Care Transition™ is undoubtedly affected by the social environment. Consideration for the psychosocial component of transition that adolescents and young adults are experiencing is imperative. Entering adulthood, there are many shifting resources and responsibilities that patients must navigate, related to: care management, financial issues, support services, care coordination, and the psychological burden this all entails. For this reason, trainees should explicitly be taught what these psychosocial issues are (Fig. 3.1) and what resources are available.

Social Differences Between Pediatric and Adult Care

	Pediatric Care	Adult Care
Care monitoring	Per guardian(s)	Per patient
Finances and insurance	Per guardian(s)	Per patient
Support services	Readily available	Not as available
Care coordination	Visits and procedures coordinated	Not necessarily

Fig. 3.1 Psychosocial variations between pediatric and adult medical care

Often, care that was previously provided and monitored by parents or guardians is now being taken on by the adolescents and young adults, and they should be supported in this process. At the same time that they are taking over their own care, young adults also are often attempting to take charge of their own finances and insurance issues for the first time. Keep in mind this is being done while support services and insurance options are both shifting for these patients with complex chronic conditions.

Additional layers are added to this psychosocial transition if there are multiple providers or specialists involved, as asynchronous transfers can occur to multiple adult physicians. This can affect multidisciplinary clinics, multidisciplinary procedures, and care coordination. Pediatric patients often have excellent care coordination and support services through a patient-centered medical home, whereas adult patients' medical homes often include primary care physicians without the same level of coordination or available support services.

Each psychosocial aspect mentioned here can be daunting to adolescents and young adults, but ultimately the transitions they are navigating within health care are only some of the many social transitions occurring around this same time period, with changes in school, work, housing, and support systems also occurring. Healthcare transition curriculum should highlight these issues, ensure trainees are aware of the obstacles and accompanying psychological burden, and arm trainees with resources to help ease the process of transition for their patients.

Cultural Transitions

In addition to the psychosocial transitions patients are overcoming, they must also navigate the "cultural" shift between pediatric and adult care models. Patients and families often report that there are differences in personalities, communication styles, and approach to patient care between pediatric and adult teams. These factors are difficult to define and objectively measure yet are critically important to transitional medicine. We describe these differences as "cultural" (Fig. 3.2). The culture of pediatric pulmonology is different from that of adult pulmonology; therefore this transition between cultures should also be addressed in the educational curriculum regarding healthcare transition. Simply put, if patients are expected to navigate this cultural shift, they need to be aware of it. In turn, if providers are expected to educate patients about this cultural shift, they too need to be aware of it.

Fig. 3.2 Cultural variations between pediatric and adult medical care

Cultural Differences Between Pediatric and Adult Care

Pediatric Pulmonology	Adult Pulmonology
Multi-disciplinary CHRONIC care	Multi-disciplinary ICU care
May serve as primary care provider	Generally not primary care provider
Often provides care most of childhood, with one primary disease process	Often treat pulmonary diseases diagnosed later in life, and in setting of other medical conditions

Pediatric pulmonology optimizes multidisciplinary care for chronic conditions in the outpatient setting and even participates in multidisciplinary procedures (e.g., ENT and pulmonology coordinating for same-day procedures in patients with cystic fibrosis). On the other hand, adult pulmonology optimizes multidisciplinary care in the intensive care unit but perhaps less effectively in the outpatient setting.

Children with chronic illnesses often have one disease process, and as such pediatric pulmonologists may serve as primary care providers for some of their long-term patients, functioning as their medical home. Adult pulmonologists do not generally serve as primary care providers, as they often care for pulmonary diseases that are one of the many comorbidities affecting their patients. In that vein, adult pulmonologists coordinate with patient-centered medical homes but are often not the primary contributors. In addition, what constitutes multidisciplinary care teams and what capabilities they possess differ between institutions, so the format and availability of resources can also be expected to change during this transfer to adult care.

Communication

An important avenue to navigating these social and cultural changes during the process of healthcare transition is effective communication. This critical phase of health care is fraught with the potential for errors stemming from miscommunication or even a lack of communication. Patients and family members deserve preparation for this transition process, and this starts first with communication.

We have a duty to prepare patients for transition in general but also specifically prepare them for the ways communication in adult medicine differs from that in pediatric medicine. A family-centered approach is used in pediatrics, with communication going through the caregiver(s). Adult medicine has the opposite approach to communication, focusing instead on the patient and their autonomy, while placing family at the periphery. In addition, pediatrics utilizes a paternalistic approach to patient care, as opposed to adult medicine where shared decision-making is prioritized, and the patient-physician relationship is viewed as a partnership.

Not only should we be preparing patients for transfer and the anticipated communication changes, but we need to communicate among healthcare teams. There are a lot of key players involved in a patient with chronic illness transitioning from pediatric to adult care, and preparation and communication are likely the best ways to minimize the risk of errors. Communication should occur between physician and patient, between physician and family members, between pediatric and adult providers, with consulting teams, and with multidisciplinary care team members to ensure aspects such as insurance, medications, and equipment are addressed. This web of communication can quickly become tangled, as shown here (Fig. 3.3), unless there is thoughtful and purposeful organization, such as can be delivered by a dedicated medical home who curates transfer packets with the pertinent medical information.

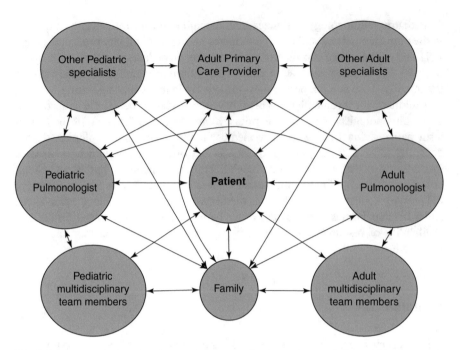

Fig. 3.3 The complexity of various active communication pathways during transition to adult care. Which pathways are emphasized or utilized most depend on the healthcare system

This degree of complexity in communication is not easy to manage, and the manner in which information is relayed varies according to healthcare system. Therefore, this is a learning opportunity for trainees. It is incumbent upon medical education training programs to be aware that the transition protocol and communication methods available at one institution do not apply to all healthcare systems, and trainees should be educated accordingly. Adult pulmonary trainees should be aware of what preparation and communication is expected in the earlier stages of transition, as this will enable them to emphasize and even clarify any confusion after the transfer to adult medicine occurs. Both adult and pediatric trainees should be educated about the nature of communication used by their counterparts, which could be leveraged on both sides to ease the shift from paternalistic conversations with caregivers to shared decision-making with young adults. In addition, if we teach patients how to be an equal partner in their care—starting in young adulthood—it makes it easier for them to become invested in the adult model of care.

Ultimately, this all is dependent upon communication. Without appropriate communication, knowledge of diseases and transition only does so much and cannot translate into improved patient care. Since it is clear that communication is convoluted during this period of transition, trainees should be given a holistic education about the transition process in order to prepare them for all variations they may encounter in practice.

Proposed Plan for Future Training

These transition topics provide a guideline for the content that needs to be included in a comprehensive curriculum for pulmonary trainees. In order to meet the needs of training programs and for the benefit of the aging pediatric population, a detailed framework should be developed. This framework should be detail-oriented enough to provide concrete direction but flexible enough to be feasible at all pulmonary training programs.

Pediatric Pulmonary Fellowship Transition Education

A model curriculum for pediatric pulmonary fellowship will include a variety of experiences that ideally will highlight all of the transition topics outlined above but also provide increased exposure to adult patients, adult pulmonary fellows and faculty, and the adult care model. Concepts of healthcare transition and adult care models should be integrated into didactics. Combined adult and pediatric transition case conferences, as well as appropriate clinical opportunities, should be made available to the fellows. Clinical experiences should include active participation in the healthcare transition process for a variety of patients, clinical exposure to a wide array of adult care models, and an optional elective in "Transitional Pulmonary Care." This multimodal approach (Fig. 3.4) increases the likelihood of a meaningful learning experience for each trainee and creates intentional educational interactions while maintaining an emphasis on experiential learning.

Adult Pulmonary Fellowship Transition Education

The model adult pulmonary fellowship curriculum would mirror the pediatric program to some degree. It would need to address healthcare transition topics, as well as increase exposure to adolescent patients, pediatric pulmonary fellows and faculty, and the pediatric care model. Like pediatric programs, the adult curriculum would include integrating concepts of healthcare transition and pediatric care models into didactics, creating combined adult and pediatric transition case conferences, and creating clinical opportunities for the fellows to experience pediatric and adolescent medicine.

However, the adult pulmonary curriculum would need to also incorporate common congenital and pediatric pulmonary diseases into their lecture curriculum, as medical knowledge in these topics is often cited as a source of discomfort or uncertainty for adult physicians [5, 6]. Clinical experiences for the adult pulmonary fellows would also need to entail inpatient and outpatient exposure to key transitional

Proposal for Transition Education in Pediatric Pulmonary Fellowship

Incorporate topics into fellowship didactics:
    concepts of transition to adult care models

- **Goal: 1-2 lectures per year**

Clinical exposure to adult care models:
    e.g., adult cystic fibrosis and pulmonary clinics, adult wards/ICU, bronchoscopy

- **Goal: patient log of 10-20 encounters**

Active participation in transition process

- **Goal: 20 patients**

Transition case conferences
    with both adult and pediatric fellows and faculty

- **Goal: 1 per year**

"Transitional Pulmonary Care" elective

- **Goal: 1 month**

Fig. 3.4 Sample curriculum for pediatric pulmonary fellowship transition education

diseases. In addition, there should be opportunities to participate in the transition process itself, albeit what this consists of would depend upon individual site availability. This could range from simply making sample transition packets available for adult pulmonary trainees, or invitations to attend meetings or calls or workgroups, or ideally even a "Transitional Pulmonary Care" elective. The adult pulmonary curriculum also utilizes a multimodal approach (Fig. 3.5) but requires a more concerted effort to fill key knowledge gaps such as those in pediatric diseases and of the healthcare transition process.

Barriers

The barriers to creating and implementing educational curriculum such as these are multifactorial. First, we know that many institutions either lack an existing transition program or the quality is not adequate [3, 4, 7, 10]. It becomes difficult to educate fellows about ideal transition programs if you do not have one available to display. However, continuing a "top-down" approach to transition preparation, where you focus on building programs and policies but neglect to educate trainees, is also inadequate. Program development without simultaneously educating our graduating workforce guarantees insufficient preparation, because the trainees of

Proposal for Transition Education in Adult Pulmonary Fellowship

Incorporate topics into fellowship didactics:
   concepts of transition AND common congenital or pediatric pulmonary diseases

- **Goal: 2-3 lectures per year**

Clinical exposure to key transitional diseases:
   inpatient and outpatient

- **Goal: patient log of 10-20 encounters**

Opportunities for adult fellows to participate in transition process

- **Goal: 3-5 patients**

Transition case conferences
   with both adult and pediatric fellows and faculty

- **Goal: 1 per year**

"Transitional Pulmonary Care" elective

- **Goal: 1 month**

Fig. 3.5 Sample curriculum for adult pulmonary fellowship transition education

today are the attendings of tomorrow as well as the medical directors and administrators in the coming years. We should be implementing and fine-tuning transition programs but also staffing these programs with physicians adequately trained in transition health care.

Furthermore, it follows that if there is a lack of quality existing transition programs, there will likely be a shortage of faculty who are qualified to teach and model transition care. There is a great need for adult and pediatric faculty and trainees who are invested in the transition process. Passionate leadership is needed to ensure educators have the resources to build curricula. Passionate educators are needed to dedicate their time and expertise to developing the curricula. Passionate program leadership is needed to locate opportunities in which to place these burgeoning curricula. Last but not least, passionate trainees are needed who see the value in learning transition processes, because adult learning theory informs that learning is optimized when the material is viewed as relevant and immediately applicable [25]. Part of the hurdle for these educators and program leadership will include time and resource management: in lieu of adding additional tasks to training programs, strategic planning can morph current encounters or educational experiences into the deliberate practice of healthcare transition.

The last broad category of barriers to implementing healthcare transition curriculum includes geographical and institutional factors. Like all big changes, there should be institutional buy-in from program leadership, department leadership, and even hospital leadership. Plus, not all training programs have close affiliation with an adult or pediatric counterpart and therefore would need to intentionally seek out these transition training opportunities.

Practical Strategies

The first practical strategy for implementing transition training is to simply have a plan. Articulating a transition training plan may be the initial step to garnering interest and buy-in from all pertinent parties. In addition, programs may need to recruit local experts with knowledge and interest in transition care. Often these local experts can be found in the fields of adolescent medicine, combined internal medicine-pediatrics, and family medicine, but expertise can be garnered in a variety of places.

Another key tactic to leverage for success is to use cystic fibrosis transition programs as models. These programs are the only current pulmonary transition protocols and as such should be used as a framework for developing and optimizing transition programs and transition curriculum.

Areas Requiring Future Attention

In order to properly implement a healthcare transition curriculum such as this, fellowship program leadership will need support. There is a role for professional societies or accrediting bodies to take on this charge, by developing education materials and setting expectations. The first step—ACGME incorporating healthcare transition into pediatric pulmonary program requirements—has occurred, but momentum must continue [17]. Another future challenge will be to develop ways of measuring the success of transition training. Being able to monitor curricular changes and measure their effects will be paramount to long-term success and iterative continual improvement.

Conclusion

As an increasing number of children with congenital or childhood-onset pulmonary diseases reach adulthood and transition to adult care, our pulmonary workforce needs to be prepared. Concerted effort needs to be made to ensure this preparation occurs. In addition to the transition protocols and continuing medical education that is already in place, it is time to develop a healthcare transition educational curriculum for our training programs. The way to ensure future success in transition programs is to begin empowering our trainees with the knowledge and skills necessary for success.

References

1. American Academy of Pediatrics, American Academy of Family Physicians, American College of Physicians-American Society of Internal Medicine. A consensus statement on health care transitions for young adults with special health care needs. Pediatrics. 2002;110:1304–6.
2. American Academy of Pediatrics, American Academy of Family Physicians, American College of Physicians, Transitions Clinical Report Authoring Group. Supporting the health care transition from adolescence to adulthood in the medical home. Pediatrics. 2011;128(1):182–200.
3. White P, Cooley W, Transitions Clinical Report Authoring Group, American Academy of Pediatrics, American Academy of Family Physicians, American College of Physicians. Supporting the health care transition from adolescence to adulthood in the medical home. Pediatrics. 2018;142(5):e20182587.
4. Mubanga N, Baumgardner DJ, Kram JJF. Health care transitions for adolescents and young adults with special health care needs: where are we now? J Patient Cent Res Rev. 2017;4(2):90–5.
5. Okumura MJ, Heisler M, Davis MM, Cabana MD, Demonner S, Kerr EA. Comfort of general internists and general pediatricians in providing care for young adults with chronic illnesses of childhood. J Gen Intern Med. 2008;23(10):1621–7.
6. Peter NG, Forke CM, Ginsburg KR, Schwarz DF. Transition from pediatric to adult care: internists' perspectives. Pediatrics. 2009;123(2):417–23.
7. Goralski JL, Nasr SZ, Uluer A. Overcoming barriers to a successful transition from pediatric to adult care. Pediatr Pulmonol. 2017;52:S52–60. https://doi.org/10.1002/ppul.23778.
8. Sadun RE, Chung RJ, Pollock MD, Maslow GR. Lost in transition: resident and fellow training and experience caring for young adults with chronic conditions in a large United States' academic medical center. Med Educ Online. 2019;24(1). https://doi.org/10.1080/10872981.2019.1605783.
9. Patel MS, O'Hare K. Residency training in transition of youth with childhood-onset chronic disease. Pediatrics. 2010;126:S190–3. https://doi.org/10.1542/peds.2010-1466P.
10. Agarwal A, Willis D, Tang X, Bauer M, Berlinski A, Com G, et al. Transition of respiratory technology dependent patients from pediatric to adult pulmonology care. Pediatr Pulmonol. 2015;50(12):1294–300. https://doi.org/10.1002/ppul.23155.
11. 2017–2018 National Survey of Children's Health. Child and Adolescent Health Measurement Initiative. Data Resource Center for Child and Adolescent Health supported by the U.S. Department of Health and Human Services, Health Resources and Services Administration (HRSA), Maternal and Child Health Bureau (MCHB). https://www.childhealthdata.org/browse/survey. Accessed 1 Dec 2019.
12. American Board of Pediatrics. Pediatric physicians workforce data book, 2018–2019. Chapel Hill, NC: American Board of Pediatrics; 2019. https://www.abp.org/sites/abp/files/workforce-data2018-2019.pdf. Accessed 1 Dec 2019.
13. American Board of Internal Medicine. Number of candidate certificates issued. American Board of Internal Medicine. 2019. https://www.abim.org/~/media/ABIM%20Public/Files/pdf/statistics-data/candidates-certified-all-candidates.pdf. Accessed 1 Dec 2019.
14. Brinn NA, Talente GM. Transitional care of children with chronic diseases. In: Pediatric hospital medicine: textbook of inpatient management. 2nd ed. Baltimore: Lippincott Williams & Wilkins; 2008. p. 733–42.
15. Accreditation Council for Graduate Medical Education. ACGME common program requirements (residency). 2019. https://www.acgme.org/Portals/0/PFAssets/ProgramRequirements/CPRResidency2019.pdf. Accessed 1 Dec 2019.
16. Accreditation Council for Graduate Medical Education. ACGME common program requirements (fellowship). 2019. https://www.acgme.org/Portals/0/PFAssets/ProgramRequirements/CPRFellowship2019.pdf. Accessed 1 Dec 2019.
17. Accreditation Council for Graduate Medical Education. ACGME program requirements for graduate medical education in pediatric pulmonology (subspecialty of

pediatrics). 2019. https://www.acgme.org/Portals/0/PFAssets/ProgramRequirements/330_PediatricPulmonology_2019_TCC.pdf?ver=2019-02-19-145146-363. Accessed 1 Dec 2019.

18. Accreditation Council for Graduate Medical Education. ACGME program requirements for graduate medical education in pulmonary disease (subspecialty of internal medicine). 2019. https://www.acgme.org/Portals/0/PFAssets/ProgramRequirements/149_PulmonaryDisease_2019_TCC.pdf?ver=2019-03-28-155735-293. Accessed 1 Dec 2019.

19. Accreditation Council for Graduate Medical Education. ACGME program requirements for graduate medical education in pulmonary disease and critical care medicine (subspecialty of internal medicine). 2019. https://www.acgme.org/Portals/0/PFAssets/ProgramRequirements/156_PCCM_2019_TCC.pdf?ver=2019-06-13-102635-373. Accessed 1 Dec 2019.

20. Accreditation Council for Graduate Medical Education. ACGME program requirements for graduate medical education in combined internal medicine - pediatrics. 2019. https://www.acgme.org/Portals/0/PFAssets/ProgramRequirements/700_InternalMedicinePediatrics_2019_TCC.pdf?ver=2019-03-26-091222-673. Accessed 1 Dec 2019.

21. Accreditation Council for Graduate Medical Education. ACGME program requirements for graduate medical education in family medicine. 2019. https://www.acgme.org/Portals/0/PFAssets/ProgramRequirements/120_FamilyMedicine_2019.pdf?ver=2019-06-13-073936-407. Accessed 1 Dec 2019.

22. Kuo AA, Ciccarelli MR, Sharma N, Lotstein DS. A health care transition curriculum for primary care residents: identifying goals and objectives. Pediatrics. 2018;141:S346–54.

23. Wright RJ, Howard EJ, Newbery N, Gleeson H. 'Training gap' – the present state of higher specialty training in adolescent and young adult health in medical specialties in the UK. Future Healthc J. 2017;4(2):80–95.

24. Got Transition™. The national alliance to advance adolescent health. https://www.gottransition.org/providers/index.cfm. Accessed 1 Dec 2019.

25. Knowles MS, Holton EF, Swanson RA. The adult learner: the definitive classic in adult education and human. 8th ed. New York: Routledge; 2015.

Part II
Psychosocial Considerations in Transition

Chapter 4
Developmental and Psychosocial Challenges for Self-Management and Maintaining Adherence to Chronic Therapies

Jennifer L. Butcher

Introduction

The transition from pediatric to adult healthcare has traditionally been conceptualized as the development of a steady progression of skills leading to independence over a predictable time period, similar to walking up a smooth slope. However, more often, the transition process is like riding an amusement park attraction, with many ups and downs, curves and bumps, and sometimes even moving backward. Although uncertainty during transition is typical, there are common areas of expected challenge. These range from broad factors related to the adolescent and young adult (AYA)'s culture and access to healthcare services, to specialized individual skills such as the ability to schedule a medical appointment. Although social-ecological and systemic factors play an important role in the transition process [1], individual factors are the best understood [2] and potentially most modifiable [3]. Chief among these individual factors are the AYA's illness self-management knowledge, skills, and behaviors [4]. This chapter provides an overview of illness self-management and its role in healthcare transition, reviews the literature on self-management within chronic lung disease, identifies developmental and psychosocial variables impacting self-management, and provides recommendations for addressing these variables and promoting self-management during care transition.

J. L. Butcher (✉)
Michigan Medicine C.S. Mott Children's Hospital, Ann Arbor, MI, USA
e-mail: jennbutc@med.umich.edu

© Springer Nature Switzerland AG 2021
C. D. Brown, E. Crowley (eds.), *Transitioning Care from Pediatric to Adult Pulmonology*, Respiratory Medicine,
https://doi.org/10.1007/978-3-030-68688-8_4

61

Models of Illness Self-Management

Pediatric illness self-management can be defined as the "interaction of health behaviors and related processes that patients and families engage in to care for a chronic condition" [4]. Many models to explain these interactions exist including those that are disease-specific [5] and those that are more inclusive, including the classic Health Belief Model [6]. This model theorizes that appropriate self-management behaviors can be predicted by an individual's *perceptions of their illness* (view of illness severity and belief in the benefits of following the healthcare plan) in comparison to their perceived *barriers* to following this plan. Although widely cited, a criticism of this model is the challenge of translating this theory into intervention [5].

In contrast, the Transtheoretical Model of Behavioral Change [7] matches intervention strategies to each stage in the model and hypothesizes that individuals move through predictable *stages of change*, similar to developmental stages, when developing behaviors to promote their health. However, this model relies on an individual's ability to control and make changes independently and does not fully take into account systemic influences that are critical during the AYA period, such as the influence of caregivers.

A more recent model of illness self-management, the Pediatric Self-Management Model [4], takes into account *systemic influences* impacting AYAs, including individual, family, and community factors; while also categorizing influences into those that are considered fairly static (socioeconomic status) and those that are more *modifiable* (psychosocial distress). Categorizing influences into those that are challenging to change versus more amenable to change makes it easier to translate this model into targeted intervention strategies.

Although these models each focus on different influences on self-management, common among them is the understanding that successful illness self-management encompasses appropriate *knowledge* of the illness, including how to navigate challenges; and the engagement in recommended self-care behaviors or *medical regimen adherence* [8]. Illness-specific knowledge is generally best conceptualized as necessary, but not sufficient, in that it is the building block for independence, but knowledge in itself typically does not lead to significant change [9]. Interventions targeting both knowledge and medical regimen adherence have, to date, shown the strongest results [9, 10]. Medical regimen adherence is often defined as the extent to which a person's behavior matches medical or health advice [11]. Along with knowledge, it is perceived as a central part of illness self-management and is a modifiable factor that is often the target of behavioral intervention [10].

Role of Illness Self-Management in Transition

Transition from pediatric to adult care is a multiyear process that is generally conceptualized as the time period when AYAs become more independent in their medical care while also receiving less support. However, this transition is often not a smooth process and, if poorly planned, can result in significant morbidity and mortality complications for the AYA [12]. Using knowledge of these potential complications, providers have developed best practices for promoting transition among individuals with chronic lung disease, including those with asthma [13], cystic fibrosis (CF) [14], and who are dependent on respiratory technology, such as receiving home ventilator support [15]. Best practice recommendations for transition specific to AYA post lung transplantation are limited [16], but best practices for transition among all solid organ transplant recipients have been developed [17].

Best practices generally stress the measurement of "transition readiness" among the AYA population [18, 19]. Illness-related "knowledge and self-management skills are the most common factors included in measures of transition readiness, suggesting a consensus regarding these issues as key contributors" [1]; thereby placing illness self-management in a central role for successful healthcare transition. To date, preliminary research has supported the role of illness self-management in the transition process. Measurement of transition readiness has been positively related to healthcare knowledge [18], self-management beliefs [20], and self-management behaviors [21]. Although there is preliminary evidence that participation in programs designed to promote transition readiness results in positive change [22], sustained evidence is lacking [23], and there are few current links between transition readiness and adult medical outcomes [22].

Role of Illness Self-Management in Chronic Lung Disease

Transition theory and preliminary evidence support the integral role that illness self-management plays in successful transition to adult care, including among those with chronic lung disease. Unfortunately, illness self-management skills are often lacking, especially during the AYA time period when medical regimen adherence is generally the poorest [24].

Among all AYAs with chronic illness, medical knowledge has been correlated with medical regimen adherence [25], but education on its own has little evidence for prompting behavior change [10]. Further, having a cognitive deficit, especially impairment in executive function skills (organization, planning, working memory), may contribute to unique barriers to developing appropriate illness-related knowledge and skills [26].

Among AYAs with chronic lung disease, medical knowledge also plays an important role in illness self-management. There is some evidence that individuals diagnosed with asthma may be at greater risk for cognitive impairment, especially among executive function skills [27]. Further, poor health literacy (understanding of healthcare information) may negatively impact the ability to use asthma knowledge [28] and has been associated with poorer physical functioning [29]. In AYAs requiring invasive or noninvasive home ventilation, there is evidence of a cognitive impact, especially among executive function skills [30–33], but there is only preliminary evidence of the relationship between these impacts and illness-related knowledge

[31]. Among individuals diagnosed with CF, there is preliminary evidence of higher rates of executive function deficit [34], but it has not been related to treatment knowledge. Although understudied, no apparent cognitive impairment has been identified in individuals that are post heart-lung transplantation [35].

Strong evidence exists supporting the prevalence and impact of poor medical regimen adherence among all AYAs with chronic illness. Recent estimates have reported that only between 10 and 35% of adolescents across chronic illness groups can be classified as adherent to their medical regimens [10]. Poor adherence is associated with numerous negative outcomes including increased healthcare use [36], and interventions that improve adherence have shown positive benefits to health [9].

Evidence of medical regimen adherence difficulties in AYAs with chronic lung disease is also strong. Among those with asthma, adolescents have been found to take <50% of prescribed doses of daily medications [37], and similar results have been found for adolescents with CF (medication possession ratios of 45–50% per pharmacy refill data) [38]. For those receiving noninvasive home ventilation, there have been mixed results from findings that only 27% use support for >3 hours to 72% using support for 8 hours [39]. The medical regimen adherence among those using invasive home ventilation is largely unknown. Finally, adherence rates among adolescents who have received lung transplantation are understudied, but a recent article using a large dataset of pediatric heart and lung transplant recipients found that physicians reported evidence of nonadherence to immunosuppressant medications at the rate of 34% [40].

According to the Health Belief Model, understanding of barriers to medical regimen adherence is key [6]. A wide range of barriers are present during the AYA period making them more susceptible to nonadherence. These include barriers related to the family system, healthcare system, and the community. During transition of care, 53% of young adults with CF were found to have a gap in care with 12% having a gap of at least 1 year [41]. Gaps in care of 1 year or more were associated with younger age at transfer and having an adult center in a different city than the pediatric center. Further, socioeconomic status (SES) may play a role as lower adherence to airway clearance in CF has been demonstrated among those with lower SES [42]. Another criterial influence on adherence during the AYA period is family, and especially caregiver, functioning. Parental depression has been associated with poorer adherence in both CF [43] and asthma [44]. Less parental supervision is related to decreased adherence in CF [45], and intervention to improve family support improved adherence in asthma [46].

Unfortunately, societal and family influences on illness self-management can be challenging to overcome. Thus, as the Transtheoretical Model of Behavioral Change suggests, focus on individual behavioral change may be an effective intervention target [7]. Although many individual factors are also largely nonmodifiable (sex, age, cognitive functioning), as the Pediatric Self-Management Model suggests, focusing intervention on modifiable factors is key [4]. Finally, Models of healthcare transition have also highlighted focus on modifiable individual characteristics such as *treatment knowledge and medical regimen adherence* [1–3]. Familiarity with typical *adolescent development* can aid in understanding of how knowledge develops over time as well as the interaction between knowledge and behavior. Further, *psychosocial distress* is a modifiable factor impacting illness self-management [10].

Adolescent Development and Illness Self-Management

Although developmental influences are largely nonmodifiable (except with time), familiarity with these influences can significantly increase understanding of the AYA and result in the development of practical intervention approaches. Physical development occurs rapidly in adolescence along with hormonal changes that can impact health functioning independently of illness self-management behaviors. For instance, earlier age at menarche has been associated with poorer adult lung function in epidemiological studies [47], and female sex hormones appear to play a role in CF pulmonary exacerbations [48]. Additionally, with rapid physical growth, appropriate drug dosing can become challenging during adolescence.

Along with physical changes, adolescents also experience cognitive changes, including the development of abstract reasoning, executive function skills, and metacognition (awareness of thought) [49]. However, these skills develop at different rates and, in certain cases, may be impeded in individuals with chronic lung disease as previously summarized. Importantly, impediments in cognitive skills have been related to worse illness self-management [26, 28, 31].

Traditional theories of adolescent development can be applied to increase understanding of how illness self-management behaviors form and change over time. Piaget's theory of cognitive development hypothesizes that adolescents move into "the formal operational stage" of cognitive development where they develop the capacity for abstract, scientific thinking [50]. During this time, adolescents begin to generate multiple solutions to problems and can solve abstract problems that they have never encountered in real life. Although there is some evidence that being in a family who is skillful at solving complex problems may aid an adolescent in adherence to a CF regimen [51], clinical interventions to improve problem-solving skills have not yet demonstrated improvement in adolescents' CF adherence [52].

It may be that the development of abstract thought initially impedes an adolescent due to negative side effects. This includes the development of argumentativeness, self-consciousness, and self-focusing [49]. Whereas during childhood, an individual with chronic lung disease might follow their treatment regimen with little resistance; in adolescence, the teen may debate a parent or question the need to complete the regimen. Additionally, self-consciousness increases in adolescence with the development of the "imaginary audience" belief where adolescents feel that they are the focus of everyone's attention [49]. This belief may result in an adolescent not wanting to disclose their illness or engage in medical care in front of others. Adolescents with CF have identified embarrassment and desire for social acceptance as barriers to adherence [53], and a study measuring asthma adherence in adolescence found that 53% of nonadherence episodes occurred while present with friends [54]. Another distorted cognition that results from self-focus is the "personal fable," where an adolescent believes that they are unique and invulnerable to the same penalties as others [49]. This has obvious consequences for illness self-management in that an individual who does not believe that nonadherence to their medical regimen will cause harm is more likely to demonstrate poor adherence. This is at the heart of the Health Belief Model [6] and may be especially relevant for treatment regimens that are burdensome [55].

Erikson's stages of psychosocial development is another classic developmental theory that can be applied to adolescent illness self-management [56]. Erikson theorized that the major personality achievement of adolescence is the development of "identity." This includes making decisions about what defines you, your values, and your life goals [49]. During this stage, adolescents move away from family and spend more time with friends, and peer support plays a central role. This has important consequences for medical regimen adherence because improved adherence in adolescence has been positively related to more parental involvement and shared treatment responsibility across a wide range of medical illnesses [10], including asthma [46] and CF [45]. In contrast, evidence whether peer support results in improved adherence has been mixed [10]. No changes in adherence to asthma controller medication were found in adolescents participating in a peer coping support group compared to the control group [57].

Although family involvement appears to play a critical role in illness self-management into adolescence, the development of supportive friendships and peer support is critical to achieving identity as theorized by Erikson [49]; and prosocial peer support may buffer against feelings of self-consciousness, indirectly promoting adherence [58, 59]. There is some evidence that individuals with chronic lung disease may have more social withdrawal and poorer friendship quality including among those with neuromuscular disease requiring home ventilation [31], CF [60], and asthma [61]. Further, peer rejection has been found to play a significant role in the increased risk for adolescent depression [62], which in itself is related to worse illness self-management [63, 64].

Psychosocial Distress and Illness Self-Management

AYA psychosocial distress is another individual variable that negatively impacts illness self-management. Although psychosocial distress is typically modifiable, an AYA's exposure to life stress or "negative life events" is not and has important long-term consequences [65]. Specifically, stress exposure has been related to poor health outcomes in asthma [66]. Further, exposure to acute stress results in physiological symptoms, such as bronchoconstriction, that can be harmful to those with lung disease [67].

Chronic stress can also contribute to internalizing symptoms, such as mood and anxiety disorders. Adolescents with chronic illness are, as a group, at higher risk for depressive and anxiety symptoms [68, 69]. Among AYAs with chronic lung disease, higher rates of anxiety and depression symptoms have been identified in those with CF [70] and asthma [71]. Much less is known about internalizing symptoms among children requiring home ventilation. Preliminary data from one study suggests that 77% of children were rated by their parents as having "excellent" or "good" emotional adjustment and 82% were "seldom" or "only sometimes" depressed, although parent-reported symptoms of depression were significantly higher among adolescents than younger children [72]. Data among children receiving lung transplant is also limited. One study examined depression symptoms among children pre- and post-heart-lung transplant. They found that 31% of children were rated above the cutoff on a depression screener pre-transplant, which was significantly higher than populations estimate, while only 13% were rated above the cutoff post-transplant [73].

Internalizing symptoms play an important role in illness self-management for individuals with chronic lung disease. The presence of these symptoms has been identified as a barrier to medical regimen adherence in CF [63] and has been associated with increased asthma symptomology [74]. However, the role of anxiety symptoms has been mixed in that some studies have shown that increased anxiety among children is related to improvements in medical regimen adherence [75], including among those with CF [76].

Similar to internalizing symptoms, the presence of externalizing symptoms (disruptive behaviors) can impact illness self-management. Rates of externalizing symptoms among those with chronic lung disease may vary by disease type, and studies are generally focused on school-aged or younger children. Among children with CF, mean externalizing behaviors have not been found to differ significantly from community samples on broad-based measures such as the Child Behavior Checklist [77]. However, children with asthma have been found to have more disruptive behaviors than community samples [78]. Further, children with more severe asthma were found to be at higher risk for oppositional behaviors into later childhood and adolescence [79]. Rates of disruptive behaviors among those requiring home ventilation and who have received lung transplantation appear to be largely unknown.

Although rates of disruptive behaviors differ among chronic illness groups, illness self-management may be problematic for those demonstrating elevations [80]. Among school-aged children with CF and asthma, child oppositional behavior was the barrier most frequently cited by caregivers as impacting respiratory treatment adherence [81]. Further, direct observation of children with CF completing respiratory treatments found that child cooperation during individual treatments was related to higher respiratory adherence rates over 3 months [82]. These preliminary findings support that disruptive behaviors may be another important psychosocial variable impacting adherence and may be a useful intervention target.

Best Practices for Assessing and Promoting Illness Self-Management in AYA

Taken together, the transition to independent illness self-management among AYA is a complex process full of potential developmental and psychosocial barriers. However, screening and assessment of these barriers, and clinical intervention focused on promoting knowledge and skill development, should be considered the best practice during the transition period [2]. Models of illness self-management suggest that key factors to the understanding of transition from pediatric to adult healthcare include recognizing that change happens in stages over time, involves systemic influences, and includes many barriers [4, 6, 7]. Further, focusing intervention on modifiable factors is optimal [4]. Models of healthcare transition suggest that aspects of illness self-management, including medical-related knowledge and medical regimen adherence, are modifiable individual influences that are crucial to optimizing transition readiness [1].

Although developmental change during adolescence is not modifiable, interventions can be tailored based on known developmental challenges for the purpose of improving knowledge and adherent behaviors. Education should be tailored based on the individual developmental level of the AYA while ensuring understanding through teach-back methods [83] and skill demonstration [84]. Further, independence and increased responsibility should not be granted based on age, but on behavior that is closely supervised by caregivers [45, 46]. Adolescent feelings of self-consciousness and the desire for increased peer engagement can be addressed through frank discussions of the adolescent's preferences regarding disclosure of illness and coaching on how to share this information [85]. An adolescent's belief in their uniqueness can be accommodated by ensuring that they are part of medical decision-making in a developmentally appropriate manner [86]. Finally, an adolescent's feeling of invulnerability can be addressed by careful screening of risk-taking behaviors [87] and ensuring that safety nets (typically caregivers) are in place while an adolescent is transitioning to independent self-management behaviors.

In contrast to developmental level, psychosocial distress in AYA is an area that is amenable to change. Empirically-supported treatment for adolescent mood and anxiety disorders includes cognitive-behavioral therapy; and treatment for disruptive behaviors includes behavioral management training and multisystemic family therapy [88]. Psychotropic medication evaluation by appropriate child pychiatric specialists should also be considered for mood and disruptive behaviors that are clinically significant [89]. Treatment of adjustment to illness and chronic life stress may include training in health promotion strategies and intervention to boost factors related to resilience [90].

Illness self-management should be routinely screened while meeting with AYAs without caregivers present. Screening should begin by assuming nonadherence and asking specific questions related to doses missed over a certain time frame. The best practice in medical regimen adherence measurement suggests that multiple methods and sources of information should be integrated, including self-report, medical variables, electronic methods if available, and co-informants such as caregivers [91]. Screening should also include assessment of common barriers such as avoidance, forgetting, and time management [92].

Depending on supports available in the clinic, optimal screening may also include screening for mood, anxiety, or behavioral disorders [93]. A number of national organizations supporting children with chronic illness recommend routine depression and anxiety screening beginning in adolescence, including the American Diabetes Association [94]; the North American Society For Pediatric Gastroenterology, Hepatology, and Nutrition [95]; and the Cystic Fibrosis Foundation [70]. The American Academy of Pediatrics also recommends depression screening in adolescence and points out that those with chronic illness, including asthma, should be considered higher risk [96].

Data obtained from screening methods can then be used to implement in-clinic interventions designed to promote AYA illness self-management behaviors. As previously reviewed, intervention should include education along with behavioral strategies. This may include reminders (including the use of technology), problem-solving, increased family involvement and monitoring, and follow-up/accountability on the part of the AYA [10]. In general, multicomponent interventions may be the most effective, although effect sizes for adherence interventions, to date, are generally small [97]. Interventions delivered in-clinic may be sufficient for some AYA, but for those that are experiencing multiple life stressors, clinically significant mood or behavioral concerns, or for whom poor illness self-management is a chronic problem, referral to a health psychologist is recommended.

Conclusion

Developmental and psychosocial challenges to illness self-management during transition are common but unique to each individual patient. Understanding of common barriers can help providers know how to screen for and address self-management challenges. Additionally, focus on ensuring illness-related knowledge and bolstering medical regimen adherence throughout childhood into early adolescence may result in a smoother transition during AYA. Adding illness self-management screening and intervention strategies into clinical care can help an AYA's transition experience to be a thrilling, but ultimately successful, ride.

References

1. Schwartz LA, Tuchman LK, Hobbie WL, Ginsberg JP. A social-ecological model of readiness for transition to adult-oriented care for adolescents and young adults with chronic health conditions. Child Care Health Dev. 2011;37(6):883–95.
2. Blum RW, Hirsch D, Kastner TA, Quint RD, Sandler AD, Anderson SM, et al. A consensus statement on health care transitions for young adults with special health care needs. Pediatrics. 2002;110:1304–6.

3. Campbell F, Biggs K, Aldiss SK, O'Neill PM, Clowes M, Mcdonagh J, et al. Transition of care for adolescents from paediatric services to adult health services. Cochrane Database Syst Rev. 2016;4:CD009794.

4. Modi AC, Pai AL, Hommel KA, Hood KK, Cortina S, Hilliard ME, et al. Pediatric self-management: a framework for research, practice, and policy. Pediatrics. 2012;129:e473–85.

5. La Greca AM, Bearman KJ. Adherence to pediatric treatment regimens. In: Handbook of pediatric psychology. 3rd ed. New York: The Guilford Press; 2003. p. 119–40.

6. Becker MH, Drachman RH, Kirscht JP. Predicting mothers' compliance with pediatric medical regimens. J Pediatr. 1972;81:843–54.

7. Prochaska, JO, DiClemente CC. The transtheoretical approach: Crossing traditional boundaries of therapy. Homewood, Ill: Dow Jones-Irwin, 1984.

8. Lozano P, Houtrow A. Supporting self-management in children and adolescents with complex chronic conditions. Pediatrics. 2018;141:S233–41.

9. Graves MM, Roberts MC, Rapoff M, Boyer A. The efficacy of adherence interventions for chronically ill children: a meta-analytic review. J Pediatr Psychol. 2010;35:368–82.

10. Hommel KA, Ramsey RR, Rich KL, Ryan JL. Adherence to pediatric treatment regimens. In: Handbook of pediatric psychology. 5th ed. New York: The Guilford Press; 2017. p. 119–33.

11. Haynes R. Introduction. In: Haynes RB, Taylor DW, Sackett DL, editors. Compliance in health care. Baltimore: John's Hopkins University Press; 1979.

12. Pai ALH, Ostendorf HM. Treatment adherence in adolescents and young adults affected by chronic illness during the health care transition from pediatric to adult health care: a literature review. Child Health Care. 2011;40:16–33.

13. Jones MR, Frey SM, Riekert K, Fagnano M, Halterman JS. Transition readiness for talking with providers in urban youth with asthma: associations with medication management*. J Adolesc Health. 2019;64:265–71.

14. Patel A, Dowell M, Giles BL. Current concepts of transition of care in cystic fibrosis. Pediatr Ann. 2017;46:e188–92.

15. Agarwal A, Willis D, Tang X, Bauer M, Berlinski A, Com G, et al. Transition of respiratory technology dependent patients from pediatric to adult pulmonology care. Pediatr Pulmonol. 2015;50:1294–300.

16. Taylor L, Tsang A, Drabble A. Transition of transplant patients with cystic fibrosis to adult care: today's challenges. Prog Transplant. 2006;16:329–34.

17. Gold A, Martin K, Breckbill K, Avitzur Y, Kaufman M. Transition to adult care in pediatric solid-organ transplant: development of a practice guideline. Prog Transplant. 2015;25:131–8.

18. Sawicki GS, Lukens-Bull K, Yin X, Demars N, Huang IC, Livingood W, et al. Measuring the transition readiness of youth with special healthcare needs: validation of the TRAQ - transition readiness assessment questionnaire. J Pediatr Psychol. 2011;36:160–71.

19. Wood DL, Sawicki GS, Miller MD, Smotherman C, Lukens-Bull K, Livingood WC, et al. The Transition Readiness Assessment Questionnaire (TRAQ): its factor structure, reliability, and validity. Acad Pediatr. 2014;14:415–22.

20. Sawicki GS, Kelemen S, Weitzman ER. Ready, set, stop: mismatch between self-care beliefs, transition readiness skills, and transition planning among adolescents, young adults, and parents. Clin Pediatr (Phila). 2014;53:1062–8.

21. Gilleland J, Amaral S, Mee L, Blount R. Getting ready to leave: transition readiness in adolescent kidney transplant recipients. J Pediatr Psychol. 2012;37:85–96.

22. Devine K, Monaghan M, Schwartz L. Transition in pediatric psychology: adolescents and young adults. In: Handbook of pediatric psychology. New York: The Guilford Press; 2017. p. 620–31.

23. Davis AM, Brown RF, Taylor JL, Epstein RA, McPheeters ML. Transition care for children with special health care needs. Pediatrics. 2014;134:900–8.

24. Masterson TL, Wildman BG, Newberry BH, Omlor GJ. Impact of age and gender on adherence to infection control guidelines and medical regimens in cystic fibrosis. Pediatr Pulmonol. 2011;46:295–301.

25. Carbone L, Zebrack B, Plegue M, Joshi S, Shellhaas R. Treatment adherence among adolescents with epilepsy: what really matters? Epilepsy Behav. 2013;27:59–63.
26. McNally K, Rohan J, Pendley JS, Delamater A, Drotar D. Executive functioning, treatment adherence, and glycemic control in children with type 1 diabetes. Diabetes Care. 2010;33:1159–62.
27. Irani F, Barbone JM, Beausoleil J, Gerald L. Is asthma associated with cognitive impairments? A meta-analytic review. J Clin Exp Neuropsychol. 2017;39:965–78.
28. Rosas-Salazar C, Apter AJ, Canino G, Celedón JC. Health literacy and asthma. J Allergy Clin Immunol. 2012;129:935–42.
29. Mancuso CA, Rincon M. Impact of health literacy on longitudinal asthma outcomes. J Gen Intern Med. 2006;21:813–7.
30. Schwengel DA, Dalesio NM, Stierer TL. Pediatric obstructive sleep apnea. Anesthesiol Clin. 2014;32:237–61.
31. Snow WM, Anderson JE, Jakobson LS. Neuropsychological and neurobehavioral functioning in Duchenne muscular dystrophy: a review. Neurosci Biobehav Rev. 2013;37:743–52.
32. Sasannejad C, Ely EW, Lahiri S. Long-term cognitive impairment after acute respiratory distress syndrome: a review of clinical impact and pathophysiological mechanisms. Crit Care. 2019;23:352.
33. Koltsida G, Konstantinopoulou S. Long term outcomes in chronic lung disease requiring tracheostomy and chronic mechanical ventilation. Semin Fetal Neonatal Med. 2019;24:101044.
34. Piasecki B, Turska-Malińska R, Matthews-Brzozowska T, Mojs E. Executive function in pediatric patients with cystic fibrosis, inflammatory bowel disease and in healthy controls. Eur Rev Med Pharmacol Sci. 2016;20:4299–304.
35. Wray J, Radley-Smith R. Beyond the first year after pediatric heart or heart-lung transplantation: changes in cognitive function and behaviour. Pediatr Transplant. 2005;9:170–7.
36. McGrady ME, Hommel KA. Medication adherence and health care utilization in pediatric chronic illness: a systematic review. Pediatrics. 2013;132:730–40.
37. Drotar D, Bonner MS. Influences on adherence to pediatric asthma treatment: a review of correlates and predictors. J Dev Behav Pediatr. 2009;30:574–82.
38. Quittner AL, Zhang J, Marynchenko M, Chopra PA, Signorovitch J, Yushkina Y, et al. Pulmonary medication adherence and health-care use in cystic fibrosis. Chest. 2014;146:142–51.
39. Amin R, Al-Saleh S, Narang I. Domiciliary noninvasive positive airway pressure therapy in children. Pediatr Pulmonol. 2016;51:335–48.
40. Killian MO. Psychosocial predictors of medication adherence in pediatric heart and lung organ transplantation. Pediatr Transplant. 2017. http://orcid.org/000.-0002-2287-9007.
41. Sawicki GS, Ostrenga J, Petren K, Fink AK, D'Agostino E, Strassle C, Schechter MS, Rosenfeld M. Risk factors for gaps in care during transfer from pediatric to adult cystic fibrosis programs in the united states. Ann Am Thorac Soc. 2018;15(2):234–40. https://doi.org/10.1513/AnnalsATS.201705-357OC.
42. Oates GR, Stepanikova I, Gamble S, Gutierrez HH, Harris WT. Adherence to airway clearance therapy in pediatric cystic fibrosis: socioeconomic factors and respiratory outcomes. Pediatr Pulmonol. 2015;50:1244–52.
43. Barker DH, Quittner AL. Parental depression and pancreatic enzymes adherence in children with cystic fibrosis. Pediatrics. 2016;137:e20152296.
44. Wood BL, Brown ES, Lehman HK, Khan DA, Lee MJ, Miller BD. The effects of caregiver depression on childhood asthma: pathways and mechanisms. Ann Allergy Asthma Immunol. 2018;121:421–7.
45. Modi AC, Marciel KK, Slater SK, Drotar D, Quittner AL. The influence of parental supervision on medical adherence in adolescents with cysticfibrosis: Developmental shifts from pre to late adolescence. Children's Health Care. 2008;37(1):78–82. https://doi.org/10.1080/02739610701766925.
46. Duncan CL, Hogan MB, Tien KJ, Graves MM, Chorney JML, Zettler MD, et al. Efficacy of a parent-youth teamwork intervention to promote adherence in pediatric asthma. J Pediatr Psychol. 2013;38:617–28.

47. Gill D, Sheehan NA, Wielscher M, Shrine N, Amaral AFS, Thompson JR, et al. Age at menarche and lung function: a Mendelian randomization study. Eur J Epidemiol. 2017;32:701–10.
48. Sutton S, Rosenbluth D, Raghavan D, Zheng J, Jain R. Effects of puberty on cystic fibrosis related pulmonary exacerbations in women versus men. Pediatr Pulmonol. 2014;49:28–35.
49. Berk LE. Development through the lifespan, 6/e © 2014. Development; 2014.
50. Inhelder B, Piaget J. An essay on the construction of formal operational structures. In: The growth of logical thinking: from childhood to adolescence. New York: Basic Books; 1958.
51. DeLambo KE, Ievers-Landis CE, Drotar D, Quittner AL. Association of observed family relationship quality and problem-solving skills with treatment adherence in older children and adolescents with cystic fibrosis. J Pediatr Psychol. 2004;29:343–53.
52. Quittner AL, Eakin MN, Alpern AN, Ridge AK, McLean KA, Bilderback A, et al. Clustered randomized controlled trial of a clinic-based problem-solving intervention to improve adherence in adolescents with cystic fibrosis. J Cyst Fibros. 2019;18:879–85.
53. Dziuban EJ, Saab-Abazeed L, Chaudhry SR, Streetman DS, Nasr SZ. Identifying barriers to treatment adherence and related attitudinal patterns in adolescents with cystic fibrosis. Pediatr Pulmonol. 2010;45:450–8.
54. Mulvaney SA, Ho YX, Cala CM, Chen Q, Nian H, Patterson BL, et al. Assessing adolescent asthma symptoms and adherence using mobile phones. J Med Internet Res. 2013;15:e141.
55. Bishay LC, Sawicki GS. Strategies to optimize treatment adherence in adolescent patients with cystic fibrosis. Adolesc Health Med Ther. 2016;7:117–24.
56. Erikson EH. Identity, youth and crisis. New York: WW Norton Company, 1968.
57. Mosnaim G, Li H, Martin M, Richardson DJ, Belice PJ, Avery E, et al. The impact of peer support and mp3 messaging on adherence to inhaled corticosteroids in minority adolescents with asthma: a randomized, controlled trial. J Allergy Clin Immunol Pract. 2013;1:485–93.
58. Janicke DM, Gray WN, Kahhan NA, Follansbee Junger KW, Marciel KK, Storch EA, et al. Brief report: the association between peer victimization, prosocial support, and treatment adherence in children and adolescents with inflammatory bowel disease. J Pediatr Psychol. 2009;34:769–73.
59. Helms SW, Dellon EP, Prinstein MJ. Friendship quality and health-related outcomes among adolescents with cystic fibrosis. J Pediatr Psychol. 2015;40:349–58.
60. Kostakou K, Giannakopoulos G, Diareme S, Tzavara C, Doudounakis S, Christogiorgos S, et al. Psychosocial distress and functioning of Greek youth with cystic fibrosis: a cross-sectional study. Biopsychosoc Med. 2014;8:13.
61. Baker SE, Niec LN, Meade J. A comparison of friendship quality and social functioning among children with perinatally acquired HIV, children with persistent asthma, and healthy children of HIV-positive mothers. J Pediatr Psychol. 2012;37:580–90.
62. Platt B, Kadosh KC, Lau JYF. The role of peer rejection in adolescent depression. Depress Anxiety. 2013;30:809–21.
63. Hilliard ME, Eakin MN, Borrelli B, Green A, Riekert KA. Medication beliefs mediate between depressive symptoms and medication adherence in cystic fibrosis. Health Psychol. 2015;34:496–504.
64. McCormick King ML, Mee LL, Gutiérrez-Colina AM, Eaton CK, Lee JL, Blount RL. Emotional functioning, barriers, and medication adherence in pediatric transplant recipients. J Pediatr Psychol. 2014;39:283–93.
65. Marum G, Clench-Aas J, Nes RB, Raanaas RK. The relationship between negative life events, psychological distress and life satisfaction: a population-based study. Qual Life Res. 2014;23:601–11.
66. Wright RJ, Cohen RT, Cohen S. The impact of stress on the development and expression of atopy. Curr Opin Allergy Clin Immunol. 2005;5:23–9.
67. McQuaid EL, Fritz GK, Nassau JH, Lilly MK, Mansell A, Klein RB. Stress and airway resistance in children with asthma. J Psychosom Res. 2000;49:239–45.
68. Pinquart M, Shen Y. Depressive symptoms in children and adolescents with chronic physical illness: an updated meta-analysis. J Pediatr Psychol. 2011;36:375–84.

69. Pinquart M, Shen Y. Anxiety in children and adolescents with chronic physical illnesses: a meta-analysis. Acta Paediatrica Int J Paediatr. 2011;100:1069–76.
70. Quittner AL, Abbott J, Georgiopoulos AM, Goldbeck L, Smith B, Hempstead SE, et al. International committee on mental health in cystic fibrosis: Cystic Fibrosis Foundation and European cystic fibrosis society consensus statements for screening and treating depression and anxiety. Thorax. 2016;71:26–34.
71. Lu Y, Mak KK, van Bever HPS, Ng TP, Mak A, Ho RCM. Prevalence of anxiety and depressive symptoms in adolescents with asthma: a meta-analysis and meta-regression. Pediatr Allergy Immunol. 2012;23:707–15.
72. Lumeng JC, Warschausky SA, Nelson VS, Augenstein K. The quality of life of ventilator-assisted children. Pediatr Rehabil. 2001;4:21–7.
73. Wray J, Radley-Smith R. Depression in pediatric patients before and 1 year after heart or heart-lung transplantation. J Heart Lung Transplant. 2004;23:1103–10.
74. Richardson LP, Lozano P, Russo J, McCauley E, Bush T, Katon W. Asthma symptom burden: relationship to asthma severity and anxiety and depression symptoms. Pediatrics. 2006;118:1042–51.
75. Wu YP, Aylward BS, Steele RG. Associations between internalizing symptoms and trajectories of medication adherence among pediatric renal and liver transplant recipients. J Pediatr Psychol. 2010;35:1016–27.
76. White T, Miller J, Smith GL, McMahon WM. Adherence and psychopathology in children and adolescents with cystic fibrosis. Eur Child Adolesc Psychiatry. 2009;18:96–104.
77. Sheehan J, Massie J, Hay M, Jaffe A, Glazner J, Armstrong D, et al. The natural history and predictors of persistent problem behaviours in cystic fibrosis: a multicentre, prospective study. Arch Dis Child. 2012;97:625–31.
78. McQuaid EL, Kopel SJ, Nassau JH. Behavioral adjustment in children with asthma: a meta-analysis. J Dev Behav Pediatr. 2001;22:430–9.
79. Goodwin RD, Robinson M, Sly PD, McKeague IW, Susser ES, Zubrick SR, et al. Severity and persistence of asthma and mental health: a birth cohort study. Psychol Med. 2013;43:1313–22.
80. Malee K, Williams P, Montepiedra G, McCabe M, Nichols S, Sirois PA, et al. Medication adherence in children and adolescents with HIV infection: associations with behavioral impairment. AIDS Patient Care STDS. 2011;25:191–200.
81. Modi AC, Quittner AL. Barriers to treatment adherence for children with cystic fibrosis and asthma: what gets in the way? J Pediatr Psychol. 2006;31:846–58.
82. Butcher JL, Nasr SZ. Direct observation of respiratory treatments in cystic fibrosis: parent-child interactions relate to medical regimen adherence. J Pediatr Psychol. 2015;40:8–17.
83. Ha Dinh TT, Bonner A, Clark R, Ramsbotham J, Hines S. The effectiveness of the teach-back method on adherence and self-management in health education for people with chronic disease: a systematic review. JBI Database System Rev Implement Rep. 2016;14:210–47.
84. Mosnaim GS, Pappalardo AA, Resnick SE, Codispoti CD, Bandi S, Nackers L, et al. Behavioral interventions to improve asthma outcomes for adolescents: a systematic review. J Allergy Clin Immunol Pract. 2016;4:130–41.
85. Venetis MK, Chernichky-Karcher S, Gettings PE. Disclosing mental illness information to a friend: exploring how the disclosure decision-making model informs strategy selection. Health Commun. 2018;33:653–63.
86. Grootens-Wiegers P, Hein IM, van den Broek JM, de Vries MC. Medical decision-making in children and adolescents: developmental and neuroscientific aspects. BMC Pediatr. 2017;17:120.
87. Klein DA, Paradise SL, Landis CA. Screening and counseling adolescents and young adults: a framework for comprehensive care. Am Fam Physician. 2020;101:147–58.
88. Christophersen ER, VanScoyoc SM. Treatments that work with children: empirically supported strategies for managing childhood problems. 2nd ed. Washington, DC: American Psychological Association; 2013.

89. Strawn JR, Dobson ET, Giles LL. Primary pediatric care psychopharmacology: focus on medications for ADHD, depression, and anxiety. Curr Probl Pediatr Adolesc Health Care. 2017;47:3–14.
90. Aujoulat I, Dechêne S, Lahaye M. Non-disease specific health promotion interventions for chronically ill adolescents in medical settings: a systematic review. Front Public Health. 2018;6:301.
91. Quittner AL, Espelage DL, Ievers-Landis C, Drotar D. Measuring adherence to medical treatments in childhood chronic illness: considering multiple methods and sources of information. J Clin Psychol Med Settings. 2000;7:41–54.
92. Quittner AL, Pedreira PB, Bernstein R, McLean LA, Nicolais CJ, Saez-Flores E, Riekert KA. Development of the adherence barriers questionnaire-cystic fibrosis (ABQ-CF): frequently endorsed barriers from openended interviews. Pediatr Pulmonol. 2016;51:465.
93. Quittner AL, Abbott J, Hussain S, Ong T, Uluer A, Hempstead S, et al. Integration of mental health screening and treatment into cystic fibrosis clinics: evaluation of initial implementation in 84 programs across the United States. Pediatr Pulmonol. 2020;55:2995–3004.
94. American Diabetes Association. Standards of Medical Care in Diabetes, 2018. Diabetes Care 2018;41(Suppl. 1).
95. Rufo PA, Denson LA, Sylvester FA, Szigethy E, Sathya P, Lu Y, et al. Health supervision in the management of children and adolescents with IBD: NASPGHAN recommendations. J Pediatr Gastroenterol Nutr. 2012;55:93–108.
96. Zuckerbrot RA, Cheung A, Jensen PS, REK S, Laraque D. Guidelines for adolescent depression in primary care (GLAD-PC): part I. Practice preparation, identification, assessment, and initial management. Pediatrics. 2018;141:e20174081.
97. Pai ALH, McGrady M. Systematic review and meta-analysis of psychological interventions to promote treatment adherence in children, adolescents, and young adults with chronic illness. J Pediatr Psychol. 2014;39:918–31.

Chapter 5
Parents in Transition: Moving from Providing to Supporting Roles

Karen Lowton

Introduction

Research examining parents' roles in their child's healthcare transition process has been conducted across a number of conditions of childhood onset including pulmonary disease. Findings identify common parental expectations, needs, challenges and concerns in supporting their children and interacting with health service professionals, with subtle differences in the family's experiences according to the impact of the underlying condition and its treatment [1]. This chapter draws on health and social science research in healthcare transition across a range of these long-term conditions to consider how parents and clinicians understand and experience changing parental roles. The chapter focuses on how parents undergo a parallel transition, from raising their child to parenting a young person, which requires subtle adjustments to their role, for example, from active to passive supervision of activities [1]. Crucially, parents remain an important and continuing resource for young people through the transition; both they and young people need coordinated attention and support from the clinical team during and after the transition process, albeit in qualitatively different ways [2].

Background

Transitional healthcare continues to be a policy priority for the growing number of children ageing with rare or complex health conditions and their care providers [3]. A successful transition is expected to produce a responsible, autonomous patient

K. Lowton (✉)
Department of Sociology, University of Sussex, Brighton, UK
e-mail: K.lowton@sussex.ac.uk

© Springer Nature Switzerland AG 2021
C. D. Brown, E. Crowley (eds.), *Transitioning Care from Pediatric to Adult Pulmonology*, Respiratory Medicine,
https://doi.org/10.1007/978-3-030-68688-8_5

who competently self-manages their condition and is ready to attend adult services in a timely fashion as the principal communicator with the adult team [4–6]. Clinicians therefore anticipate that during transition young people will take on 'a more empowered and active role as independent adult healthcare consumers' [4], seceding responsibility for their own healthcare from their parents' oversight.

Clinicians initially assumed that young people's needs during transition could be addressed solely by structural and procedural changes to healthcare systems and services [5], framing parents as people who need to be 'educated' to 'step back' and 'let go' [4]. An assumption that all elements of the young person's development (e.g. cognitive, emotional, physical and psychosocial) occurred at the same pace led to an anticipation of transition being a linear process. Clinicians' conceptualisation of parental care and involvement was largely binary; parents were essential in caring for all their child's needs, but a young person no longer required parental support. As such, clinicians supposed parents held an 'emeritus' carer status once their children had left paediatric care [7] and in early transition programmes ongoing parental input was largely positioned as problematic.

Perhaps as a result of clinicians' assumptions about them, parents worried that their child's transition to adult services would not allow them to be as involved in their care as they were previously [8]. Parents reported feeling ignored or sidelined at this point [9] with minimal clinical understanding of how they experienced the transition process in the context of their own needs. As Allen et al. [10] note, it was ironic that support for parents was often withdrawn at the very time when their needs for professional support and information were high. The small amount of research and service evaluation conducted at this time therefore neglected to capture a complete picture of young people and their families in transition [11], focusing instead on the 'experiences' of small samples, with little research including parents' perspectives [1, 12]. Even at the beginning of this century, there was scant evidence of the impact of healthcare transition on families [4], although there was an emerging recognition that families could become 'partners' in the transition process if they were sufficiently prepared.

Problematising the 'Family'

Parents provide support that all adolescents need to become more skilled at managing their own lives and together with the wider family are a key source of support for young people [13]. Rather than treading a short and linear path to independence in adulthood, young people tend to live for longer in their parental homes in most developed countries [13] and continue to experience a strong bond with their families after leaving home [14]. Even in the context of 'healthy' young people, the assumption of a smooth trajectory towards independence has ignored the individual and changing nature of parental relationships and their importance for young people [13], leading to the nature of relationships between young people and their families more generally being under-investigated [15]. However, regardless of clinical and societal expectations of autonomy, individuality and independence [13], it is vital to consider the family structures and practices, including support, resources and contact, that each young person draws on through their transition. Of course, young people may live with one or more parents, in blended or extended families, experiencing different family values, communication styles and socio-economic status. In this chapter, acknowledging the heterogeneity of families, the term 'parent' is used to describe any adult that has significant responsibility for providing care and protection for a child or young person.

Early assumptions are now being surpassed by a growing acknowledgement that it is the family rather than the individual patient that is key to a successful transition to adult care. Just as an artificial distinction exists between 'child' and 'young person', so too exists an artificial distinction between parents caring and ending care for their child post-paediatric care; it is erroneous to think that families will 'let go', 'step back' or 'give up' [4] all the caring roles they enacted when their children were young. Strategies for improvements in the transition process increasingly recognise parents as an important component of successful transition through enabling their child to assume increasing responsibility for their health, providing a protective factor for their wellbeing and teaching their child skills necessary to self-manage their condition [11]. Transition should therefore be understood as a process involving an adaptation in care roles for both patients and parents. Views of both young people and their parents were considered in developing the UK's NICE guideline for improving care during transition [16], yet there is limited evidence to guide healthcare professionals as to what constitutes 'effective' parenting in transition and how they can support parents as they modify their roles [17], although early work provides many useful ideas.

The Nature of Paediatric Care and the Long-Term Condition

The philosophy of transition care is at odds to that of paediatric care, which works from a family systems approach to ensure that, as primary caregivers, parents are significantly involved in negotiating, advocating and making health-related decisions for their child [2]; for some parents their role will take a substantial portion of their time and form a significant part of their identity. In this environment, parental security is established through good working relationships with paediatric teams and from the continuity of their child's care that subsequently develops [12]. Over time, parents learn how to navigate the paediatric system, experience working in partnership with professionals, with their opinions largely being sought and welcome [6].

Two groups of young people essentially transition out of paediatric care: one with relatively stable and 'minimal' disease that can relatively easily leave behind their parents' involvement in their care routines and one that will have ongoing need for parental support through transition and into adult care, due to complex, progressive and unpredictable disease trajectories and health needs. The latter group, the focus of this chapter, needs to not only maintain daily control of their health by mastering complex symptom management but also learn to communicate directly with health professionals about their symptoms and care needs and manage their clinic appointment schedules. There is a risk for parents of these young people to feel that their achievements made in paediatric care will be lost at transition, with little opportunity to build new relationships with clinicians and a sense of sorrow or abandonment at no longer being needed in the same way.

Historically, many parents (and their clinicians) delayed their child leaving paediatric care due to the absence of transition services and the lack of adult physicians trained to treat young people with complex conditions of childhood onset [4]. Cultural gaps in consulting styles between paediatric and adult clinicians were also slow to be addressed and communicated to families [12]. This reluctance to leave paediatric care may indeed have contributed to adult clinicians' perceptions of parents needing to 'let go' of their child and no longer be the decision-makers for their child's care [11].

Below I set out the key concerns that parents anticipate and experience at their child's move to transition care before focusing on their worries about the young person specifically.

What Are Parents' Key Concerns at the Time of Their Child's Transition?

Concerns About Post-paediatric Care Services

Limited awareness of the standard and availability of post-paediatric services continues to underlie many parents' feelings of being unprepared or unable to anticipate how their child's future needs will be met by healthcare services [1, 11]. For some, this perceived lack of preparation together with a lack of communication may lead to feelings of abandonment by healthcare professionals [1], concerns of whether transition will happen at the 'right time' for their child [12] and increasing uncertainty, ambivalence and reluctance to begin handing over care responsibilities to the young person [18].

For other parents, post-paediatric services are seen as complex, confusing, fragmented and procedural, leading to feelings of 'falling off a cliff' [19], their child being a 'number' on a 'conveyor belt', and perceptions of a lack of consistency in staff approaches [17]. For example, parents express concern that clinicians will neither realise that a young person is a new patient and give appropriate support nor establish relationships with families of young patients in transition [12, 20]. Others report a sense of disillusionment with health and social care systems that fail to meet the full range of families' complex needs [6, 21].

Through these concerns, parents have two key difficulties. First is anticipating the health-specific challenges ahead: both service-focused (such as where and from whom future care will be delivered) and the quality of that care [8]. Second is protection of their child which is an issue of highest concern to parents [17], with threats arising not only from their health condition and uncertainty around future morbidity and mortality but also from more general worries about what is to come [2], including social and cultural issues such as sexual activity and employment opportunities. Transition care does not always respond to all the needs of young people, who also experience the broader and more typical transitions and anxieties during adolescence such as experiencing sexual relationships, managing self-confidence, leaving education, starting work or higher education and perhaps moving away from the family home. Here, clinicians should not only consider risks and uncertainties but also wider vulnerabilities to ensure a holistic approach [17].

Concerns About the Young Person

Many parents want to retain a sense of control of their child's health condition even when the young person with a rare or complex condition is an adult [12]. In that sense, they are not so unlike parents of 'healthy' young people who remain mindful of their child's ongoing health status and behaviour. Parents appear pivotal in developing their children's decision-making abilities, especially in challenging times [22]. Although a range of studies note the anxiety, uncertainty and fear that many parents experience at the time of their child's transition, these emotions may not commonly be expressed to healthcare professionals because parents are concerned about not being seen as over-advocating for their child or being 'difficult', as well as unfamiliarity with who and how they should express their concerns [21]. However parental anxiety can have a negative impact on the transfer of care tasks to the child and potentially lead to parents' overprotection of their child [18]. No relationship has yet been identified between parental anxieties and particular patient profiles [8]; thus developing more individualised patient transition protocols remains problematic.

Aware that their experience has been built over years, parents may also believe their child is unable to grasp and competently manage complex care in transition [23] or be ready to conduct all care tasks independently [4, 8]. Thus, parents may express concerns about a handover of care responsibility within a relatively short timeframe and at a challenging point in their child's life course. Perceived lack of adequate transition care may lead parents to continue as the care coordinator, assuming responsibility for communicating between different services and scheduling appointments [1]. Additionally, young people may decide not to seek healthcare during their adolescent years, there being a difference between capacity for independent action and making the choice to do so [10]. 'Control' or overprotection and conflict with young people over parents' 'constant checking' and questioning have been reported as children become more proficient at managing (or neglecting) their own care [1]. However, despite expressing ongoing worries and their need to plan, parents also report working to adopt a balanced approach to their child's care that is not too restrictive or permissive [17].

It is relatively easy for parents to transfer routine and straightforward tasks, such as medication-taking, but harder to hand over responsibility for more complex tasks such as coordinating different care providers and decision-making for complex symptoms [17]. Parent's handing over of care roles is therefore complex and requires delicate support to achieve a balance. For instance, parents' desire to protect the young person's long-term wellbeing, for example, in nurturing their independence in self-management, can conflict with their need to protect their immediate health, especially for conditions that are unpredictable and potentially life-threatening [17] or where symptoms such as breathlessness mean parents need to access formal care on the young person's behalf [17, 23, 24].

For young people with rare conditions, care challenges also relate more widely to the lack of public understanding of what it is like to experience a particular condition and how this might impact how a young person experiences their daily life [23]. Parents' continuing concerns around the potential exclusion of their child from elements of social life have been noted [2], even when robust transition processes are in place. Parents of young people who are 'behind' in developing their social skills also need careful acknowledgement and support [17]. In these cases, parents' extended roles reflect quite reasonable responses to their child's social precarity [17].

Parents therefore remain key role models for their children, actively exposing them to opportunities where they can learn, enhance and display their self-care abilities in safe environments with increasing confidence [17]. Supporting families to cope with these very real worries appears to be a vital part of effective transition care [17]. The following section outlines some ideas for supporting parents.

Suggestions

Timing of Transition

Young people enter and move through transition services in relation to their own and their parents' changing roles and relationships. There are therefore no 'one size fits all' approach to successful healthcare transition and no evidence that young people's transition to self-management will continue at the same pace at home as in the clinic. Parents usually have a good understanding of when their child is ready to enter a transition programme, for example, through their increasing maturity, sense of responsibility, emotional stability and capacity to self-manage their condition [1], yet families still need time to adjust to the idea of transition. Planning discussions should begin at an early point in the process to give young people and their families in paediatric care time to adjust. As their child matures, parents do make alterations to their caring roles including their responsibilities, decision-making and healthcare management [11]. Across a number of more recent studies, parents have been noted to perceive the transition towards their child's self-management as important, generally positive and something that young people are motivated to do, facilitated by parents gradually 'upskilling' the young person towards that goal [1]. The timing of healthcare transition therefore needs to be flexible, occurring when the young person and their parents feel it is appropriate and taking parents' concerns and suggestions into account [6]. Parents also need to be able to assure themselves that their child's transition programme is high-quality and comprehensive and has a similar intensity of care to the paediatric service the family is leaving behind while understanding that the style of care their child receives will be qualitatively different [4].

Providing Information

Parents receiving information at the same time as their child can help in numerous ways, for example, to enable them to feel prepared, informed, involved and reassured; to feel more secure when their child has left paediatric care; to help avoid misunderstandings about care intentions; and to facilitate future family and professional discussions [12]. Well-informed and confident parents are likely to be better equipped to pass on their knowledge and experience to support the young person's self-management skills [25]. Both preparatory and ongoing conversations and information are required [11], ensuring that transition care is not only in place but is visible to the family. General information about how transition and adult care is organised, including location, appointment format and clinic location, is essential [12]. However, information may be confusing and irrelevant, lack important detail or sometimes be too much in volume for parents to be able to filter what is immediately relevant to their child [2]. In communicating with young people and their parents, clinicians need to think not only about what information needs to be conveyed but also what form it will take [12], for example, a series of written plans that the young person and their parents can refer back to over time. Alongside this information, how their child will receive essential information such as what they should do if they become ill, or prepare for travelling, is also valued [12]. Parents' input into a transition plan that is then written for the young person may help to reassure the family that key information has not been forgotten [12].

A separate meeting for parents to meet the new clinicians should be an explicit part of the transition process preparation plan [8, 12], with the paediatric team introducing the patient and their family to the adult team [4]. Clinicians' collaboration with parents before the transition process begins can help establish their relationship with the new care team generally [12]; it is also helpful to identify a healthcare professional specifically responsible for providing care to the young person. For instance, a named coordinator, key worker or 'navigator' can be assigned to support the young person and their parents through the transition programme. This individual can identify and relay appropriate information at key time points, get to know the family [2, 5], communicate with the wider healthcare team [6] and be a specific resource for the young person [5].

Enabling Network Support

Establishing a forum for parents and young people to share their experiences outside transition clinic appointments is an innovative way to support families. For example, peer support groups for young people with similar conditions could provide a network for their child to share their experiences and may help to allay parents' concerns that their child may be socially isolated [12]. Parental peer support groups in paediatric care can also enable parents to have a greater understanding of the extent of planning required for transition and the need for young people to begin to take ownership, developing a sense of belonging and mutual support and empowerment for parents and young people alike [21]. The shared experiences noted in research with parents of young people already in transition programmes with a range of underlying diagnoses suggest that non-disease-specific interventions for parents may help support their own role transition [1]. For example, parents may be able to gain new knowledge and became more future-oriented and active in preparing for transition [21] and their child's increasing responsibilities more generally. Peer parental support groups in transition can also enable parents to share their experiences, facilitate discussion of risky health behaviours and collectively problem-solve challenges such as how they could respond to the young person [12] and garner ideas for future planning [21]. Through parents meeting parents of older children, experiences of how other young people were able to take on more responsibility over time, and the benefits and challenges of this, can also be learned [12]. However, much peer support research to date in this context has involved small samples and pilot interventions, with high non-attendance rates at support groups due to competing demands on parents' time. Encouraging time-pressured parents to draw on a trusted network of supports outside their family such as teachers and peers at school may also help to support parents in their changing roles [1].

Communicating with Young People

It is vital to explain the rationale for developmentally appropriate transition care and have early and open discussions with parents about it – for example, where and when lone consultations with the young person will occur and who sets the pace and agenda of these [10]. Health professionals' belief that parents gradually lose their right to information about the young person has historically been embedded in their practice [24]. Similarly, many young people will anticipate attending transition clinic appointments alone but that their parents will continue to provide support and advice at home [10, 24]. Transition clinicians are required to simultaneously respect the young person's autonomy and confidentiality while involving and supporting their parents so that they feel secure that their child's care needs are being met [12] and that they could meet their child's future needs if called upon to do so (e.g. in periods of acute illness). The extent of trust that parents have in their child's transition team underpins many of their beliefs about the appropriateness of maintaining the confidentiality of their child [26]. If the transition service does offer lone consultation, it is crucial to think about who sets the pace of this; early conversations with the young person and their parents about their preferred styles of consulting can help inform how consultations are patterned. Whatever the consulting arrangements, parents should continue to have access to practical advice and support regarding caring for their child [10], and be kept informed about issues they need to be aware of, within the limits of confidentiality. Parents may triangulate clinical advice with different sources of information and their own instinct [23]; talking to parents about other sources of ideas and how that might affect their ideas and experience of the transition process may help to avoid misunderstandings and stresses.

Confidential care is just as important for young people with a rare or complex condition as for those who are healthy [27]. Confidential consultations enable clinicians and patients to discuss more sensitive issues [4] and address young people's more typical health concerns. In the context of chronic illness, both parents and young people report healthcare professionals having good listening skills, being honest and maintaining confidentiality, as important [28]. Conversely, evidence also suggests a degree of parental involvement in care leads to improved health outcomes [1]. Parents identify both a range of benefits and harms of confidential care which may reflect a more general conflict associated with parenting any adolescent [29]. Complexity and controversy therefore surround lone consulting and confidentiality both for transition staff and parents, for example, what should be done if the young person has not attended their appointments and there is concern about their health, if parents believe young people are hiding vital concerns from clinicians or if the team senses that parents may be reading the young person's private clinic correspondence. The importance young people place on confidentiality may prevent them attending transition appointment if they sense a risk of their parents receiving or passing on their private information, yet complete exclusion of parents is difficult, especially if they believe their child is not coping [12].

In working to resolve concerns of confidentiality, it may be possible for clinicians to consider a longer appointment once a year for children around 12 years and over, the first part of which is a lone patient consultation, accompanied by provision of information about this format to young people and their parents [27]. In thinking about the limits of maintaining confidentiality, confidentiality may be better understood as a continuum than a binary [29], whereby three distinct options for disclosure outside the consultation are available on a spectrum between the two extremes of breaching and maintaining confidentiality: where the young person decides to disclose; where the professional discloses with permission of the young person; and where the professional breaks confidentiality with the young person's knowledge but not consent. Here, understanding the young person's issue and their developing autonomy can be considered. However, dilemmas of confidentiality involve weighing multiple and conflicting risks with immediate and future harms, and professionals are unlikely to agree limits to confidentiality in all cases. Duncan et al. [29] list a range of strategies that can be used to minimise the potential for harm when managing confidentiality with young people: conducting thorough risk assessments; maintaining the therapeutic relationship; empowering the young person; supporting the whole family; and professional safety. This approach to conceptualising confidentiality highlights the complexity that needs to be worked through with young people and their parents.

Supporting the Parental Role

Parents should be understood as a resource for both the young person and healthcare team, with their expertise being acknowledged and taken into account in care planning [12]. Transition programmes must therefore include the family [4], recognising that parents are likely to have a continuing and adapting supportive role in providing care for the young person that might never be discontinued. Parental support appears to be a key factor in encouraging and facilitating young people to understand and build their ability to self-manage their condition [30] such that they become experts in their own care [1]. Being instrumental in their child's transition, parents remain active in preparing them for adult care, for example, by increasing the range and type of care tasks the young person undertakes and by moving to 'shared care' within the home [1]. It is useful therefore to consider parents as an integral part of the young person's supportive healthcare team and transition care for a young person as 'shared care' between the healthcare team and parents. Professional care needs to be directed towards both the young people and their parents in achieving this, developing transition programmes and service structures that recognise and respond to the continuing caring role played by parents [10], even as this role qualitatively changes as the young person grows older.

Parental involvement in transition care is a delicate and ongoing balance [29]. Ambiguity and uncertainty abound over what transition and adult care arrangements signify about parents' changed role, for example, their previous 'management' role may give way to a 'consultant' or supervisory one [1, 9, 24]. Working to allay parental anxieties will help parents feel supported in gradually handing over care tasks to their child. Identifying and addressing their concerns regarding risk, uncertainty and vulnerability can equip parents and young people to manage better through, for example, problem-solving, communication skills and role clarification [17]. Throughout the transition process, clinicians should regularly ask young people whether and how they would like to involve their parents in their care and in what capacity they should be communicated with [16]. While the young person is living in the family home and with the young person's permission, it is reasonable for clinicians to take advice from parents about their child and incorporate relevant points into ongoing transition care planning and to keep the parents broadly informed of plans when there are issues of which the family need to be aware [10].

Many of parents' initial concerns can be ameliorated if clinicians check in with parents once transition of care is underway [8].

Healthcare professionals are more likely to gain support from parents through building rapport and communicating the rationale and importance of care that appropriately addresses all aspects of the young person's wellbeing [17, 27]. However, just as care for the young person needs to be individualised, profession-als' support for parents also needs to focus on their specific needs as their role in formal services and at-home shifts [12], understanding the stresses and challenges associated with changes at transition, including feelings of loss around the ending of the relationship with healthcare providers [11].

Working Towards Independence

Independence and autonomy are best understood as gradual, incremental and nego-tiated processes, with parents gradually transferring responsibility for self-care, in accordance with other increasing responsibilities, to their child, for example, in education and employment [1]. Parental care can be considered as a continuum or hierarchy of tasks and involvements; some are easily transferred as the child grows older (e.g. taking daily medication), whereas others (e.g. driving a young person to their appointments when this is the preferred option for the family) may be negoti-ated within the family and continue long into adulthood. Nevertheless, evidence consistently suggests transition is a complex and 'messy' process, with multiple transitions occurring for the young person and their family [10]. Clinicians should not assume that there will be an equivalent or smooth pace of transition to indepen-dence and autonomy in the home environment and should consider how cultural differences may influence the autonomy of young people in self-managing their condition. Most families work through their own processes of transferring care tasks, recognising differences in capacity and choice, and healthcare systems should be there to support them in this. Similarly, although 'independence' may apply to clinic visits and some care tasks, 'interdependence' may be a more realistic way of understanding a young person's care transition within the family home [31].

The process of young people assuming responsibility from their parents is part of a child's normal development but for young people with rare and complex condi-tions is often more challenging. As each child matures, parents make alterations to their caring roles including their responsibilities, decision-making and healthcare management [11]. Young people may also push back at parents for more control of their own care yet default back to them in times of acute illness. Roles and respon-sibilities therefore change differently over time as children become less reliant on their parents; some will be taken over gradually with parental supervision, for example, scheduling and ordering medication doses, where others may continue to be primarily held by parents, for example, advocating for a critically ill young per-son [24]. Others may be learnt in transition, for example, arranging clinic and refer-ral appointments. Young people in private/insurance healthcare systems may need extra parental support here, for example, in finding appropriate insurance policies and understanding reimbursement and associated bureaucratic elements [4]. For some tasks a young person will self-initiate taking responsibility, for others their parent may be explicit in transferring responsibility, or indeed the process of transferring responsibility for a care task may occur in response to an unforeseen event [32]. Role realignment is therefore generally renegotiated, with changes being instigated by both parents and young people [17].

In reality, full responsibility may be the aspiration, but this is less clear when parents remain involved in managing at least some aspects of the young person's care. Few explicit discussions about responsibilities or what 'full responsibility' might entail [32] typically occur, and due to a host of reasons, the young person may move backwards and forwards in taking on responsibilities. With development of a young person's independence and autonomy, the definition of a 'successful' self-management may be negotiated. Here clinicians need to be aware that not complying with a treatment plan may be a young person's active choice [4], even though health outcomes may be adversely impacted [33]. Responsibility for care might also return to the parents if the young person disengages from transition process or needs respite care in periods of extreme illness or if end of life care is needed. Parents will struggle to catch up with immediate care needs they are expected to provide if they have had no involvement with professionals over many years. It is also important to be aware of a reverse protectionism that can occur in more complex and life-limiting conditions whereby the young person seeks to shield their parents from news about their deteriorating health state [24, 31].

Conclusion

Transition teams work to fit young people and their parents into an existing healthcare system and service ethos, albeit a relatively new one. To facilitate their gradual handing over of responsibility for care tasks to their child and collaborate with healthcare professionals in efforts to transfer care tasks, parents need to be prepared for transition, informed and involved. Support strategies need to recognise the diversity of family experiences, goals and complex health conditions. Secure and consistent relationships between professionals, parents and young people appear likely to enable parents to be a steady resource and source of support.

Responsibility for care needs to be transferred incrementally at a reasonable pace, despite the change of venue and teams being swift. Parents and young people have many complex needs during healthcare transition that are not yet fully appreciated nor understood by clinicians and researchers [11]. The process of supporting both young people and their parents through transition is a balancing act, with teams having to navigate carefully between supporting both sets of needs [12]. Being aware that families have their own ways of managing transition away from the clinic, providing support and avoiding a prescriptive 'one size fits all' appears to offer a pragmatic way through the transition process.

More focused, higher-quality research is required with larger, more culturally diverse samples that take the unique context of each family into account [11]. Well-defined intervention studies, with evaluation of both effectiveness and family experiences, would aid understanding of how best to support families in transition. Additionally, more nuanced work focusing on how young people's condition-specific and developmental changes impact their parents as they grow older will also enable more specific guidance to be given.

References

1. Heath G, Farre A, Shaw K. Parenting a child with chronic illness as they transition into adulthood: a systematic review and thematic synthesis of parents' experiences. Patient Educ Couns. 2017;100(1):76–92.
2. Björquist E, Nordmark E, Hallström I. Parents' experiences of health and needs when supporting their adolescents with cerebral palsy during transition to adulthood. Phys Occup Ther Pediatr. 2016;36(2):204–16.
3. van Staa A, Jedeloo S, van Meeteren J, Latour JM. Crossing the transition chasm: experiences and recommendations for improving transitional care of young adults, parents and providers. Child Care Health Dev. 2011;37(6):821–32.
4. Rosen DS. Transition of young people with respiratory diseases to adult health care. Paediatr Respir Rev. 2004;5(2):124–31.
5. Rapley P, Davidson PM. Enough of the problem: a review of time for health care transition solutions for young adults with a chronic illness. J Clin Nurs. 2010;19(3–4):313–23.
6. Davies H, Rennick J, Majnemer A. Transition from pediatric to adult health care for young adults with neurological disorders: parental perspectives. Can J Neurosci Nurs. 2011;33(2):32–9.
7. Ross HM, Fleck D. Clinical considerations for allied professionals: issues in transition to adult congenital heart disease programs. Heart Rhythm. 2007;4(6):811–3.
8. Boyle MP, Farukhi Z, Nosky ML. Strategies for improving transition to adult cystic fibrosis care, based on patient and parent views. Pediatr Pulmonol. 2001;32(6):428–36.
9. Lowton K. Parents and partners: lay carers' perceptions of their role in the treatment and care of adults with cystic fibrosis. J Adv Nurs. 2002;39(2):174–81.
10. Allen D, Channon S, Lowes L, Atwell C, Lane C. Behind the scenes: the changing roles of parents in the transition from child to adult diabetes service. Diabet Med. 2011;28(8):994–1000.
11. Betz CL, Nehring WM, Lobo ML. Transition needs of parents of adolescents and emerging adults with special health care needs and disabilities. J Fam Nurs. 2015;21(3):362–412.
12. Bratt EL, Burström Å, Hanseus K, Rydberg A, Berghammer M, On behalf on the STEPSTONES-CHD consortium. Do not forget the parents—Parents' concerns during transition to adult care for adolescents with congenital heart disease. Child Care Health Dev. 2018;44(2):278–84.
13. Wyn J, Lantz S, Harris A. Beyond the 'transitions' metaphor: family relations and young people in late modernity. J Sociol. 2012;48(1):3–22.
14. Heath S, Cleaver E. Young, free and single?: twenty-somethings and household change. Basingstoke: Palgrave Macmillan; 2003.
15. Gillies V. Young people and family life: analysing and comparing disciplinary discourses. J Youth Stud. 2000;3(2):211–28.
16. NICE Guideline. Transition from children's to adults' services for young people using health or social care services. 2016. https://www.nice.org.uk/guidance/ng43/evidence/full-guideline-pdf-2360240173. Accessed 1.11.2020.

17. Shaw KL, Baldwin L, Heath G. 'A confident parent breeds a confident child': understanding the experience and needs of parents whose children will transition from paediatric to adult care. J Child Health Care. 2020; https://doi.org/10.1177/1367493520936422.
18. Sable C, Foster E, Uzark K, Bjornsen K, Canobbio MM, Connolly HM, et al. Best practices in managing transition to adulthood for adolescents with congenital heart disease: the transition process and medical and psychosocial issues: a scientific statement from the American Heart Association. Circulation. 2011;123(13):1454–85.
19. Joly E. Transition to adulthood for young people with medical complexity: an integrative literature review. J Pediatr Nurs. 2015;30(5):e91–e103.
20. Burström Å, Öjmyr-Joelsson M, Bratt EL, Lundell B, Nisell M. Adolescents with congenital heart disease and their parents: needs before transfer to adult care. J Cardiovasc Nurs. 2016;31(5):399–404.
21. Kingsnorth S, Gall C, Beayni S, Rigby P. Parents as transition experts? Qualitative findings from a pilot parent-led peer support group. Child Care Health Dev. 2011;37(6):833–40.
22. Carr-Gregg M, Enderby K, Grover S. Risk-taking behaviour of young women in Australia: screening for health-risk behaviours. Med J Aust. 2003;178:601–4.
23. Kayle M, Tanabe P, Shah NR, Baker-Ward L, Docherty SL. Challenges in shifting management responsibility from parents to adolescents with sickle cell disease. J Pediatr Nurs. 2016;31(6):678–90.
24. Iles N, Lowton K. What is the perceived nature of parental care and support for young people with cystic fibrosis as they enter adult health services? Health Soc Care Community. 2010;18(1):21–9.
25. Ford CA, Davenport AF, Meier A, McRee AL. Partnerships between parents and health care professionals to improve adolescent health. J Adolesc Health. 2011;49(1):53–7.
26. Sasse RA, Aroni RA, Sawyer SM, Duncan RE. Confidential consultations with adolescents: an exploration of Australian parents' perspectives. J Adolesc Health. 2013;52(6):786–91.
27. Duncan RE, Jekel M, O'Connell MA, Sanci LA, Sawyer SM. Balancing parental involvement with adolescent friendly health care in teenagers with diabetes: are we getting it right? J Adolesc Health. 2014;55(1):59–64.
28. Farrant B, Watson PD. Health care delivery: perspectives of young people with chronic illness and their parents. J Paediatr Child Health. 2004;40(4):175–9.
29. Duncan RE, Hall AC, Knowles A. Ethical dilemmas of confidentiality with adolescent clients: case studies from psychologists. Ethics Behav. 2015;25(3):197–221.
30. Kirk S, Beatty S, Callery P, Gellatly J, Milnes L, Pryjmachuk S. The effectiveness of self-care support interventions for children and young people with long-term conditions: a systematic review. Child Care Health Dev. 2013;39(3):305–24.
31. Lahelma E, Gordon T. Resources and (in (ter)) dependence: young people's reflections on parents. Young. 2008;16(2):209–26.
32. Nightingale R, McHugh G, Kirk S, Swallow V. Supporting children and young people to assume responsibility from their parents for the self-management of their long-term condition: an integrative review. Child Care Health Dev. 2019;45(2):175–88.
33. Sawyer S, Drew S, Yeo M, Britto M. Adolescents with a chronic condition: challenges living, challenges treating. Lancet. 2007;369:1481–9.

Chapter 6
Using a Social-ecological Framework to Guide Transition

Pi Chun Cheng, Michael M. Rey, Dava Szalda, and Lisa A. Schwartz

Introduction

The Maternal and Child Health Bureau and National Alliance to Advance Adolescent Health's "Six Core Elements of Health Care Transition," built from the consensus guidelines of the American Academy of Pediatrics and other societies, emphasize the importance of a formalized transition process for adolescents and young adults (AYA) that includes repeated assessment of transition readiness [1]. Nevertheless, until recently there has been little consensus on how to define the components of transition readiness and how to appropriately evaluate it. A framework for transition readiness that is founded in theory and validated was needed.

Pi Chun Cheng and Michael M. Rey contributed equally with all other contributors.

P. C. Cheng
Division of Pulmonary Medicine, Children's Hospital of Philadelphia, Philadelphia, PA, USA
e-mail: chengp1@email.chop.edu

M. M. Rey (✉)
Division of Pulmonary, Allergy, & Critical Care Medicine, University of Pennsylvania and University of Pennsylvania Perelman School of Medicine, Philadelphia, PA, USA

Division of Pulmonary and Critical Care Medicine, Corporal Michael J. Crescenz VA Medical Center, Philadelphia, PA, USA
e-mail: michael.rey@pennmedicine.upenn.edu

D. Szalda · L. A. Schwartz
Division of Oncology, Children's Hospital of Philadelphia and University of Pennsylvania Perelman School of Medicine, Philadelphia, PA, USA
e-mail: szaldad@email.chop.edu; schwartzl@email.chop.edu

© Springer Nature Switzerland AG 2021
C. D. Brown, E. Crowley (eds.), *Transitioning Care from Pediatric to Adult Pulmonology*, Respiratory Medicine,
https://doi.org/10.1007/978-3-030-68688-8_6

The Social-ecological Model of AYA Readiness to Transition (SMART) was developed by Schwartz and colleagues to fill this gap [2]. Built on theoretical models including social-ecological models of adaptation and disease management, the SMART model provides a framework for transition, identifying aspects of transition readiness that include both objective, difficult to change pre-existing factors and also subjective, modifiable variables. In this chapter we will define the SMART model, its components, validation, and general use. To show the way that the SMART model can be incorporated into transition in respiratory disease, we will then briefly apply it to the transition literature for pulmonary and respiratory diseases including cystic fibrosis, chronic respiratory failure in neuromuscular disease, asthma, and pulmonary hypertension.

SMART Model

The SMART model builds upon the social-ecological framework that places the AYA at the center of a series of inter-related perspectives – of patients, families, and healthcare providers – and the reciprocal relationships that develop therein. These perspectives and relationships are in turn impacted by larger systems that can include cultural influences, social networks, healthcare policies, and political influences. Relying on this structure, the model acknowledges that two separate patients, for example, may be of the same age and disease profile but have very different levels of transition readiness. For example, the patient's individual personality and experience, their family, their providers, their relationships with those family members and providers, their culture, and their communities may influence their readiness for transition and, as a result, their outcomes through that transition. It is only through awareness of this larger social-ecological context that the transition readiness can be understood. In addition to this understanding, the model also provides an opportunity to assess readiness across these domains to allow for interventions that can be studied and implemented.

Through this theoretical framework, the SMART model identifies 11 components of readiness to transition [2]. Four components are pre-existing factors. These are objective factors that are difficult to modify and, therefore, less amenable to intervention. These are (1) sociodemographics/culture, (2) access/insurance, (3) medical status and risk, and (4) neurocognition/IQ. There are also seven subjective factors that are modifiable and more amenable to intervention. Six of these apply to patients, caregivers, and healthcare providers. These include (1) knowledge, (2) skills/self-efficacy, (3) beliefs/expectations, (4) goals/motivation, (5) relationships/communication, and (6) psychosocial/emotions. The seventh, developmental maturity, is specific to patients. The description of these components is adapted from Schwartz et al.'s initial articulation in 2011 [2].

Objective Components

The objective components of transition readiness identified by the SMART model are pre-existing factors that impact patients, parents, and providers. These are difficult to change but can influence the stakeholders to transition both directly and indirectly through their impact on the subjective components.

Sociodemographics and culture include patient age, gender identity, ethnic and racial identity, socioeconomic status, and the culture of the patient, family, and community. It is expected that older age and higher socioeconomic status and a culture that positively views or affects healthcare access and transition are facilitators of the transition process. Each of these aspects will in turn influence all other components of transition readiness.

Access and insurance include the availability of adequate insurance to cover needed services and treatments, ability to pay for cost-sharing, and access to medical providers capable of caring for the particular healthcare needs of the AYA. Even patients with adequate insurance that is continuous through the transition period may have difficulty finding adult providers who are comfortable and capable of caring for AYA with special healthcare needs. Gaps in any of these aspects will serve as barriers to the transition process and transition readiness.

A patient's diagnosis, disease history, and the particular complications or future risks serve as the foundation for *health status and risk*. These aspects are the care needs entailed by the disease itself. Rarer diseases that require pediatric expertise or individuals with unique aspects to their disease presentation and management may have additional barriers to transition when compared to other AYA with healthcare needs.

Lastly, unlike knowledge or developmental maturity, *neurocognitive status/IQ* is thought to be challenging to change. Intact neurocognition and at least average IQ serve as facilitators, whereas cognitive impairment and intellectual disability may serve as barriers to transition readiness and the transition process.

Subjective Factors

Unlike the objective aspects underlying transition readiness, the subjective factors are more modifiable. Through repeated assessments, evaluations, and interventions, these will change over time and as such may serve as ideal targets for interventions to improve transition readiness. With the exception of *developmental maturity*, which applies only to patients and highlights a patient's developing autonomy and outgrowing the family-oriented pediatric healthcare setting, the other subjective components apply equally to patients, families, and providers. Readiness on the part of all parties is needed to facilitate successful transition.

Whereas health status/risk refers to the actual health history and risks of future complications, *knowledge* is the patient's, family's, and provider's understanding of that history and health status and needs. It necessitates that participants, including both pediatric and adult providers, know the pertinent details of the patient health history. All must also recognize the importance and benefits of transition. This factor can be facilitated by the formalization of the introduction of a transition process and the maintenance of a transition health summary as outlined in the American Academy of Pediatrics guidelines on transition and the Six Core Elements of Health Care Transition [1, 3].

Skills and self-efficacy relate to the ability to manage personal health, health care, and the transition itself. This may include scheduling appointments, ordering medication refills, and/or ensuring follow-through on treatment plans. This is among the most studied and evaluated aspect of transition for AYA with special healthcare needs. It also serves as the target of one of the more studied and utilized transition readiness assessments, the Transition Readiness Assessment Questionnaire (TRAQ) [4–8]. These assessments, however, typically focus primarily on the patient and ignore the provider and the family. Providers and caregivers also require skills in helping to coach, guide, and prepare the patient for transition. Examples of collaborative skills include shared decision-making and responsibility and navigating the adult healthcare system from the perspective of referring provider, or patients and parents.

This highlights a number of other subjective factors that influence transition. *Goals and motivation* reference the importance that patients, providers, and family share the same goals through the transition process. Transition is facilitated by shared interest in developing patient self-management skills and shared goal to move to adult care. *Relationships and communication* between all groups, including both pediatric and adult providers, should be collaborative, clear, and geared toward supporting health and transfer of care. Absence of shared goals to develop patient independence and dependent relationships such as that of the parent and AYA may be barriers to transition. Underlying this are the *beliefs* and expectations related to the transition process. All need to believe that the transition process is important and will be positive for the patient in the long run. Such a belief can build long-term trust in the healthcare system and establish a foundation for continued engagement in care.

Lastly, *psychological functioning or emotions* highlight the way that psychological conditions and emotions surrounding the transition process can serve as either facilitators or barriers. A family functioning well and coping appropriately with life stress, parties that are psychologically well and not dealing with crises, and individuals that feel confident, prepared, and empowered can help to support transition. Transitioning during a time of heightened psychological stress and conflict or fear and anxiety about the transition process may make transfer at that time more challenging. Additionally, recognition and management of co-occurring mood disorders including anxiety and depression for patients and families is important in facilitating transition.

Validation

The validity of the SMART model and its 11 components of transition readiness have been established in the years since its introduction. Surveys, focus groups, and interviews have been conducted with providers, families, and AYA with special healthcare needs [2, 9]. Through these, stakeholders both supported the components and their definitions and also reported differing opinions in what they perceived to be the most important components [9]. This suggests that the model is applicable and comprehensive while also validating the need for perspectives of multiple stakeholders. Further, the Transition Readiness Inventory (TRI), a transition readiness assessment built on the SMART model foundation, has also recently been developed and validated in survivors of childhood cancer [10]. Unlike other transition readiness assessments, the TRI is a multi-informant assessment with both parent and patient versions [10, 11]. The content validity was determined by multiple stakeholders including providers, patients, and parents further lending support for the underlying model that serves as its theoretical basis [10].

The validity of the SMART model has been further supported as the model has been incorporated into the transition literature of multiple different patient populations. Again, surveys and interviews with stakeholders in the care of patients with sickle cell disease, survivors of childhood cancer, inflammatory bowel disease, and type 1 diabetes, have lent support to the multi-informant components of the SMART model to a variety of disease states [12–16]. This suggests that the model is broadly applicable to transitioning AYA.

The SMART model has not been directly validated in pulmonary patient populations but was described as a framework for transition in cystic fibrosis [17, 18]. Nevertheless, as the transition process is being investigated in pulmonary and respiratory disease, many of these same themes and components emerge. As with the other health conditions in which it has been studied, a social-ecological model such as SMART is incredibly applicable to pulmonary diseases. Pulmonary diseases that affect AYA may require regular follow-up and reassessment of disease state, complex management regimens, and multiple provider types. Additionally, across disease states there is wide variability in disease severity and outcomes, changes in disease course through adolescence, and pediatric provider experience that may not be as readily available with adult providers. The SMART model would, then, serve as an effective framework and tool by which to assess and improve transition readiness in pulmonary disease. We now turn to an investigation of the SMART model though transition in pulmonary disease.

SMART in Pulmonary Disease

Cystic Fibrosis

Cystic fibrosis (CF) has, in many ways, served as the model for a traditionally pediatric disease that has become a pediatric and adult disease and for which a transition process is important. Over 30,000 individuals in the USA and more than 70,000 worldwide have CF, an autosomal recessive disease in which the CFTR protein, an ion channel found in tissues across organ systems, is aberrant [19]. Through scientific and care advancements, survival has increased dramatically, and a remarkable demographic shift has occurred. By 2018, in just 40 years, CF had gone from a disease with only 10% of affected individuals aged 18 years or older to one in which 55% of patients are adults [19]. Survival is only expected to continue to improve as new drugs that target the underlying molecular mechanism are now available to 90% of patients with CF [19]. Transition to adult care has, then, become a necessity in CF care.

In addition to the changes in survival, the complexity of CF and its management highlights the importance of a model such as SMART in transition management. Though the morbidity and mortality are due primarily to pulmonary disease, the ubiquity of the CFTR protein across organ systems makes CF a multi-system disease. In addition to lung disease, patients have sinus disease, luminal and liver gastrointestinal disease, nutritional deficiencies, endocrinopathies, joint disease, and higher rates of anxiety and depression [19]. Each of these may require a separate medical specialist to aid in management. Additionally, the pulmonology office typically serves as the medical home, seeing patients quarterly and coordinating this care. While this role may be common in pediatrics, it is unusual in adult subspecialty care outside of CF care. The adult CF center had to be built to be such a medical home. For patients and their families, the daily care can be equally intensive; it requires a median of seven medications and taking over 1.5 hours for treatments [20]. Readiness for transition on the part of patients, families, and providers, then, is also paramount to facilitate the needed transition.

Applying the SMART model to the extant CF transition literature and practices can highlight not only the ways in which such a framework is already in use but also how it could be utilized in a more comprehensive fashion to assess and improve readiness for patients. Transition in CF has often recognized the importance of multiple stakeholders – patients, families, and providers – to effective transition. In an effort to both emphasize the importance of transition as a goal and also to prepare adult providers to care for patients with CF, the CF Foundation, a national advocacy organization that accredits the CF care centers where the majority of patients with CF receive their care, has mandated that centers provide care in an adult-oriented model and has funded the training of adult providers in the care of patients with CF [21–23]. They additionally provide support materials geared to patients and families to teach and prepare for transition.

In addition, a number of objective, pre-existing factors have been identified as impacting the efficacy of transition and transition readiness for patients with CF. Sociodemographics, insurance status, and ease of access to providers, for example, have been associated with prolonged gaps in care, classified as greater than 365 days between the last encounter at a pediatric center and the first at an adult center [24]. Younger age at time of transition, lack of health insurance, and transfer to an adult center in a different city than the pediatric program were associated with such prolonged gaps [24]. Similarly, health status has been identified as an influencer of the perception of readiness to transfer. A survey of pediatric and adult CF providers identified medical severity as a barrier to transfer, with patients perceived to be sicker having a delayed transition process [22].

The CF transition literature has also identified a number of the subjective, modifiable components outlined by the SMART model as components of transition. As in other conditions, much of this work, to date, has focused on the patient and assessing patient knowledge, skills, and efficacy [18]. Two validated CF-specific transition readiness assessments have been created that primarily assess these domains [11]. Additionally, both the TRAQ and a modified caregiver version of the TRAQ have also been used in CF transition care. Perceptions of readiness for self-care differed between patients and caregivers, highlighting the importance of multi-informants advocated by the SMART model and the role for interventions to target both patients and parents [25]. Even these multi-informant assessments, however, focus almost solely on disease management skills [25]. Still, across this work, older age and structured transition programs that either utilize readiness assessments or formalize transition teaching are associated with an increase in disease management skills, increased self-care, and self-advocacy skills [25, 26].

These are not, however, the only domains that have been identified and assessed in the CF transition literature. Qualitative studies and surveys of patients, family members, and providers regarding perceptions of transition have identified the importance of the patient-provider relationship, parent-child relationship, beliefs about transition, patient independence, and the goals of transition [26–28]. Structured transition programs that have been described in the literature, guidelines, and position papers from field experts emphasize the role of developing a relationship with both pediatric and adult providers, the gradual introduction and building of skills and knowledge, the early introduction of the transition to build belief in the process and to establish transition as a goal [26, 29–32].

While these individual components have been identified, the comprehensive model incorporating all is often absent. The SMART model could serve as a foundation for a fuller assessment that could be used to study both extant transition programs and to design new interventions. Fully validating this model with regard to the CF population should be undertaken, and longitudinal assessments based on the same are required. Still, the rigorous evaluation of transition for CF patients remains far ahead of many other respiratory illnesses.

Neuromuscular Disease

Progressive neuromuscular diseases (NMD), such as Duchenne muscular dystrophy (DMD), spinal muscular atrophy, cerebral palsy, and spinal cord injury, may lead to chronic respiratory failure due to weak respiratory muscles and resultant chronic hypoventilation. As in CF, advances in medical care, in particular improved respiratory support through mechanical ventilation and targeted molecular therapies, have led to marked improvement in survival with young adults now living to adulthood. For DMD, among the most common and severe forms of NMD, the mean age of survival has increased from teenage years in the 1960s to well into the 30s today [33, 34]. There is a vital and growing need to bridge pediatric to adult pulmonary care for these individuals. However, the transition process for patients with NMD has unique challenges.

Using the SMART model to assess the transition to adult care for patients with NMD and chronic respiratory failure highlights some particular challenges that may serve as barriers to transition readiness. From a neurocognitive standpoint, in addition to their physical limitations, many NMD patients also have intellectual disabilities – they may depend on their caregivers for decision-making. Lack of access to adult medical care is one of the primary barriers in the transition for NMD. There are few adult pulmonologists and institutions that are trained and well supported to care for this patient population [35]. Most young adults with NMD that lack access to appropriate adult care are still under the care of their pediatric providers. The adult providers that are available are typically at academic centers; therefore, visits may require long-distance travel – a particular challenge for this population who may require wheel chairs, are reliant on battery-powered ventilators, and need caregivers to assist with many physical needs. For those individuals lost to pediatric care, they often reengage with the medical community only in times of emergency and respiratory crisis, resulting in poor health outcomes.

Further implicating the role of access and medical status for patients with NMD, the transition from pediatric to adult care settings often comes with changes in insurance coverage, durable medical equipment companies, nursing care, and access to community resources. Simultaneous transition across these domains leads to vulnerabilities in care continuity and successful transition. The adult system is often structured differently as well. The multidisciplinary clinics where multiple specialists can evaluate a child in the same day, common in pediatrics, are rarely seen in adult practices.

Beyond the barriers in the objective factors, further examination of transition through the SMART framework also identifies several additional key factors that may initially make transition readiness more complicated in this population. For most young people, transition is a time when independence and autonomy are developing. For a young adult with a progressive neuromuscular condition, however, this is also the period in which they may face greater health decline, lose strength and mobility, and actually physically depend more on their caregivers. This loss of independence adds additional complexity in their transition process. The patient may be ready, developmentally, to build their skills and self-efficacy but must rely on others to provide medical treatments, adequate and safe housing, transportation, healthcare financing, and even avenues to socialization.

As NMD patients become increasingly physically dependent on others, many do not feel the need to develop age-appropriate disease knowledge or management skills or even to participate actively in their decision-making on their health. Young adults are often surprised by the level of disease knowledge and self-advocacy expected by their adult medical providers [36]. Some have difficulty transitioning from a family-centered pediatric care culture to individual-centered adult medical care. As a result, they may develop distrust for adult providers as their needs from the medical team are not being "met" due to different expectations. In addition, many individuals with NMD can experience social isolation, anxiety, and depression due to their declining health and inability to perform daily tasks and achieve personal goals [37, 38]. If unrecognized, mental disorders can become a significant obstacle to transition [39].

For patients and families, the emotional burden of leaving the pediatric medical team who they believe have been instrumental in managing the complexities of NMD may pose distress. Families may resist the idea of transition to adult care and may not share the goal or belief that transition and an adult-oriented system is good for their child. Pediatric providers may share the belief that adult pulmonologists are not prepared to care for patients with NMD [35]. Lastly, transition may be as difficult for the caregivers as it is for the young adults. Due to the physical limitations of patients, many caregivers provide complete care while balancing jobs to afford medical expenses. Over time, the stress of being the primary caregiver can lead to significant emotional distress and the need for respite [39, 40].

The many potential barriers and pitfalls to a successful transition for patients with NMD and chronic respiratory failure highlight the need for a comprehensive transition framework such as the SMART model. A focus on skills and efficacy alone would make for an inadequate transition process. Instead, an understanding of the social-ecological context in which the patient is situated is essential. Specifically, improving transition is dependent on training of adult pulmonologists to provide competent NMD care, changing the structure of adult care, advocating for changes to insurance policies, and improving access to assistive technologies. Even before these changes in objective factors occur, though, repeated SMART-informed assessments of all stakeholders should be used to identify areas for intervention in the subjective factors. Future clinical and research efforts should use such a model to guide and evaluate interventions to improve transition for patients with NMD and chronic respiratory failure.

Asthma

In contrast to CF and respiratory failure due to neuromuscular disease, asthma is among the most common chronic conditions in children, AYA, and adults. Twenty-five million people, or nearly 8% of the US population, and five million children under 18 have been diagnosed with asthma [41]. Perhaps because of its relatively high prevalence, 85% and 86% of surveyed primary care internists and pediatricians, respectively, reported feeling comfortable treating asthma [42]. Although there is widespread comfort in management of asthma by providers across the age span, asthma does appear to manifest differently at different ages, to have variable courses through adolescence, and thus to have different treatment plans in pediatric and adult medicine [43, 44].

Despite, or maybe because of, the frequency of asthma diagnoses and its variable course, there has been little research on transition of patients with asthma specifically and none that have looked at the readiness of the family or provider [45]. The need for transition readiness assessment and transition processes, however, remains. As with all AYA, this can be a high-risk time where individuals engage in more risk-taking behaviors. Of particular concern in the asthma population is initiation of or exposure to cigarette smoking and/or vaping. Medication adherence, loss to follow-up, and development of other comorbidities such as obesity and mental health disorders that often occur during young adulthood may also be of concern. In a randomized trial of transfer of asthma care to an adult provider, comparing transfer to an asthma specialist vs. to a primary care doctor, there were no differences in primary outcomes for patients with mild/moderate asthma based on the type of provider to whom they transferred care. Across all provider types, however, an association between bronchial hyper-reactivity and medication adherence was seen [46]. Additionally, weight gain and decreased exercise, both known risk factors for an increase in asthma symptoms, also occurred at time of transfer, again regardless of provider type [46]. On the individual level, this is a period when transition readiness assessments and processes may help to optimize outcomes through the transition.

Research to date suggests the applicability of the SMART model to asthma. Scal and colleagues showed that insurance and access to care are issues as AYA age, with young adults aged 18–24 having greater gaps in recommended care due to financial barriers, including lack of insurance, when compared to adolescents aged 12–17 [47]. A qualitative study of AYA with severe asthma asked patients to evaluate their experience with transition [48]. Among the themes that emerged were the need to take more responsibility for their care, needing themselves and not just their parents to be involved in their care, and feeling isolated, left out, and unengaged with the adult healthcare system [48]. These interviews highlighted many of the same components of transition readiness in the SMART model – the need for all parties to build skills/efficacy, the importance of strong and open relationships, and the need for an acknowledgment on the benefits and goals of transition.

Much work remains to be done in understanding specific barriers and facilitators to transition in asthma. In particular, at this time, enlarging the perspective to better understand the role of families and providers in readying for transition will be important. The incorporation of the SMART model in future research and interventions will serve to create a comprehensive and measured process.

Pulmonary Hypertension

As with asthma, pulmonary hypertension (PH) has been understudied from the perspective of transition from pediatric to adult care. While some of the underlying diseases that may cause pulmonary hypertension, namely, congenital heart disease and sickle cell disease, have been a focus of transition research, the pulmonary hypertension itself is rarely discussed. Nevertheless, the applicability of the SMART model can be seen in PH care. An educational piece in Advances in Pulmonary Hypertension, the official Advances in Pulmonary Hypertension Association an advocacy organization for patients with PH, adapted guidelines and research from other chronic disease to transition in PH [49]. They advocate for a process that incorporates many aspects of the SMART model including multiple perspectives – patients, peers, families, providers – and outline a process to identify and improve many of the subjective factors identified in the SMART model [49]. These include assessing patient development, patient and caregiver mental health, belief and knowledge, and self-efficacy among others [49].

Additionally as complex treatment regimens, including continuous parenteral therapies, have become available to children, the care of PH has become more complex but also has begun to resemble adult care more closely [50, 51]. Building readiness on the part of all stakeholders will be important to facilitate successful transition. Using the SMART model to design, assess, and revise a model of transition such as the one outlined by the Pulmonary Hypertension Association could serve as the basis of an effective transition process in this setting.

Conclusion

Transition is a dynamic, multifactorial process involving multiple stakeholders and psychosocial variables. A social-ecological framework allows for a comprehensive approach to address the different components and complex intricacies that occur in transition of care from pediatric to adult health system. We introduce SMART as a model that utilizes this theoretical framework and apply it to various respiratory conditions. As SMART was originally validated with childhood cancer survivors – a heterogeneous group with a range of symptoms and severity – so, too, are patients with respiratory conditions. As such, the multi-dimensional and multi-stakeholder nature of SMART lends itself well to respiratory diseases as it can account for major variations in transition readiness needs and factors. Future research is needed to validate the use of SMART in chronic respiratory diseases, and longitudinal and multi-site collaborations are needed to develop evidence-based interventions to improve transition of care in the field of pulmonary medicine.

References

1. National Alliance to Advance Adolescent Health. Six core elements of health care transition. gottransition.org. Accessed 12/6/2019.
2. Schwartz LA, Tuchman LK, Hobbie WL, Ginsberg JP. A social-ecological model of readiness for transition to adult-oriented care for adolescents and young adults with chronic health conditions. Child Care Health Dev. 2011;37(6):883–95. https://doi.org/10.1111/j.1365-2214.2011.01282.x.
3. White PH, Cooley WC, Transitions Clinical Report Authoring Group, American Academy of Pediatrics, American Academy of Family Physicians, American College of Physicians. Supporting the health care transition from adolescence to adulthood in the medical home. Pediatrics. 2018;142(5) https://doi.org/10.1542/peds.2018-2587. Epub 2018 Oct 22. doi: e20182587 [pii].
4. Sawicki GS, Lukens-Bull K, Yin X, et al. Measuring the transition readiness of youth with special healthcare needs: validation of the TRAQ – transition readiness assessment questionnaire. J Pediatr Psychol. 2011;36(2):160–71. https://doi.org/10.1093/jpepsy/jsp128.
5. Wood DL, Sawicki GS, Miller MD, et al. The transition readiness assessment questionnaire (TRAQ): its factor structure, reliability, and validity. Acad Pediatr. 2014;14(4):415–22. https://doi.org/10.1016/j.acap.2014.03.008.
6. Sawicki GS, Kelemen S, Weitzman ER. Ready, set, stop: mismatch between self-care beliefs, transition readiness skills, and transition planning among adolescents, young adults, and parents. Clin Pediatr (Phila). 2014;53(11):1062–8. https://doi.org/10.1177/0009922814541169.
7. Gray WN, Holbrook E, Morgan PJ, Saeed SA, Denson LA, Hommel KA. Transition readiness skills acquisition in adolescents and young adults with inflammatory bowel disease: findings from integrating assessment into clinical practice. Inflamm Bowel Dis. 2015;21(5):1125–31. https://doi.org/10.1097/MIB.0000000000000352.
8. Jensen PT, Paul GV, LaCount S, et al. Assessment of transition readiness in adolescents and young adults with chronic health conditions. Pediatr Rheumatol Online J. 2017;15(1):70–6. https://doi.org/10.1186/s12969-017-0197-6.
9. Schwartz LA, Brumley LD, Tuchman LK, et al. Stakeholder validation of a model of readiness for transition to adult care. JAMA Pediatr. 2013;167(10):939–46. https://doi.org/10.1001/jamapediatrics.2013.2223.
10. Schwartz LA, Hamilton JL, Brumley LD, et al. Development and content validation of the transition readiness inventory item pool for adolescent and young adult survivors of childhood cancer. J Pediatr Psychol. 2017;42(9):983–94. https://doi.org/10.1093/jpepsy/jsx095.
11. Schwartz LA, Daniel LC, Brumley LD, Barakat LP, Wesley KM, Tuchman LK. Measures of readiness to transition to adult health care for youth with chronic physical health conditions: a systematic review and recommendations for measurement testing and development. J Pediatr Psychol. 2014;39(6):588–601. https://doi.org/10.1093/jpepsy/jsu028.
12. Mulchan SS, Valenzuela JM, Crosby LE, Diaz Pow Sang C. Applicability of the SMART model of transition readiness for sickle-cell disease. J Pediatr Psychol. 2016;41(5):543–54. https://doi.org/10.1093/jpepsy/jsv120.
13. Szalda D, Piece L, Brumley L, et al. Associates of engagement in adult-oriented follow-up care for childhood cancer survivors. J Adolesc Health. 2017;60(2):147–53. https://doi.org/10.1016/j.jadohealth.2016.08.018.
14. Paine CW, Stollon NB, Lucas MS, et al. Barriers and facilitators to successful transition from pediatric to adult inflammatory bowel disease care from the perspectives of providers. Inflamm Bowel Dis. 2014;20(11):2083–91. https://doi.org/10.1097/MIB.0000000000000136.
15. Pierce JS, Aroian K, Schifano E, et al. Health care transition for young adults with type 1 diabetes: stakeholder engagement for defining optimal outcomes. J Pediatr Psychol. 2017;42(9):970–82. https://doi.org/10.1093/jpepsy/jsx076.
16. Cadogan K, Waldrop J, Maslow G, Chung RJ. S.M.A.R.T. transitions: a program evaluation. J Pediatr Health Care. 32(4):e81–90. https://doi.org/10.1016/j.pedhc.2018.02.008.

17. Tuchman LK, Schwartz LA, Sawicki GS, Britto MT. Cystic fibrosis and transition to adult medical care. Pediatrics. 2010;125(3):566–73. https://doi.org/10.1542/peds.2009-2791.
18. Kreindler JL, Miller VA. Cystic fibrosis: addressing the transition from pediatric to adult-oriented health care. Patient Prefer Adherence. 2013;7:1221–6. https://doi.org/10.2147/PPA.S37710.
19. Cystic Fibrosis Foundation. Cystic fibrosis foundation patient registry 2018 data report. Cystic Fibrosis Foundation. 2019.
20. Sawicki GS, Sellers DE, Robinson WM. High treatment burden in adults with cystic fibrosis: challenges to disease self-management. J Cyst Fibros. 2009;8(2):91–6. https://doi.org/10.1016/j.jcf.2008.09.007.
21. McLaughlin SE, Diener-West M, Indurkhya A, Rubin H, Heckmann R, Boyle MP. Improving transition from pediatric to adult cystic fibrosis care: lessons from a national survey of current practices. Pediatrics. 2008;121(5):e1160–6. https://doi.org/10.1542/peds.2007-2217.
22. Flume PA, Anderson DL, Hardy KK, Gray S. Transition programs in cystic fibrosis centers: perceptions of pediatric and adult program directors. Pediatr Pulmonol. 2001;31(6):443–50. https://doi.org/10.1002/ppul.1073. [pii].
23. Flume PA, Taylor LA, Anderson DL, Gray S, Turner D. Transition programs in cystic fibrosis centers: perceptions of team members. Pediatr Pulmonol. 2004;37(1):4–7. https://doi.org/10.1002/ppul.10391.
24. Sawicki GS, Ostrenga J, Petren K, et al. Risk factors for gaps in care during transfer from pediatric to adult cystic fibrosis programs in the United States. Ann Am Thorac Soc. 2018;15(2):234–40. https://doi.org/10.1513/AnnalsATS.201705-357OC.
25. Lapp V, Chase SK. How do youth with cystic fibrosis perceive their readiness to transition to adult healthcare compared to their caregivers' views? J Pediatr Nurs. 43:104–10. https://doi.org/10.1016/j.pedn.2018.09.012.
26. Coyne I, Sheehan AM, Heery E, While AE. Improving transition to adult healthcare for young people with cystic fibrosis: a systematic review. J Child Health Care. 2017;21(3):312–30. https://doi.org/10.1177/1367493517712479.
27. Iles N, Lowton K. Young people with cystic fibrosis' concerns for their future: when and how should concerns be addressed, and by whom? J Interprof Care. 2008;22(4):436–8. https://doi.org/10.1080/13561820801950325.
28. Corman LA. Factors that are associated with readiness to transition from pediatric to adult health care in cystic fibrosis: The Eberly College of Arts and Sciences at West Virginia University; 2014.
29. Okumura MJ, Ong T, Dawson D, et al. Improving transition from paediatric to adult cystic fibrosis care: programme implementation and evaluation. BMJ Qual Saf. 2014;23 Suppl 1:i64–72. https://doi.org/10.1136/bmjqs-2013-002364.
30. Chaudhry SR, Keaton M, Nasr SZ. Evaluation of a cystic fibrosis transition program from pediatric to adult care. Pediatr Pulmonol. 2013;48(7):658–65. https://doi.org/10.1002/ppul.22647.
31. Towns SJ, Bell SC. Transition of adolescents with cystic fibrosis from paediatric to adult care. Clin Respir J. 2011;5(2):64–75. https://doi.org/10.1111/j.1752-699X.2010.00226.x.
32. Bryon M, Madge S. Transition from paediatric to adult care: psychological principles. J R Soc Med. 2001;94 Suppl 40:5–7.
33. Kohler M, Clarenbach CF, Bahler C, Brack T, Russi EW, Bloch KE. Disability and survival in Duchenne muscular dystrophy. J Neurol Neurosurg Psychiatry. 2009;80(3):320–5. https://doi.org/10.1136/jnnp.2007.141721.
34. Panitch HB. 15 - Children dependent on respiratory technology. In: Kendig & Chernick's disorders of the respiratory tract in children. 8th ed; 2012. p. 261–71. http://www.sciencedirect.com/science/article/pii/B9781437719840000152. https://doi.org/10.1016/B978-1-4377-1984-0.00015-2.
35. Agarwal A, Willis D, Tang X, et al. Transition of respiratory technology dependent patients from pediatric to adult pulmonology care. Pediatr Pulmonol. 2015;50(12):1294–300. https://doi.org/10.1002/ppul.23155.

36. Abbott D, Carpenter J, Bushby K. Transition to adulthood for young men with Duchenne muscular dystrophy: research from the UK. Neuromuscul Disord. 2012;22(5):445–6. https://doi.org/10.1016/j.nmd.2012.02.004.
37. Lindsay S, McAdam L, Mahendiran T. Enablers and barriers of men with Duchenne muscular dystrophy transitioning from an adult clinic within a pediatric hospital. Disabil Health J. 2017;10(1):73–9. doi: S1936-6574(16)30138-8 [pii].
38. Bushby K, Finkel R, Birnkrant DJ, et al. Diagnosis and management of Duchenne muscular dystrophy, part 1: diagnosis, and pharmacological and psychosocial management. Lancet Neurol. 2010;9(1):77–93. https://doi.org/10.1016/S1474-4422(09)70271-6.
39. Hull J, Aniapravan R, Chan E, et al. British thoracic society guideline for respiratory management of children with neuromuscular weakness. Thorax. 2012;67 Suppl 1:1. https://doi.org/10.1136/thoraxjnl-2012-201964.
40. Nereo NE, Fee RJ, Hinton VJ. Parental stress in mothers of boys with Duchenne muscular dystrophy. J Pediatr Psychol. 2003;28(7):473–84. https://doi.org/10.1093/jpepsy/jsg038.
41. National Center for Health Statistics. National Asthma Data; National Health Interview Survey, CDC. Compiled 12/7/2020; https://www.cdc.gov/asthma/nhis/2019/data.htm. Last accessed 2/24/2021.
42. Okumura MJ, Heisler M, Davis MM, Cabana MD, Demonner S, Kerr EA. Comfort of general internists and general pediatricians in providing care for young adults with chronic illnesses of childhood. J Gen Intern Med. 2008;23(10):1621–7. https://doi.org/10.1007/s11606-008-0716-8.
43. Fuchs O, Bahmer T, Rabe KF, von Mutius E. Asthma transition from childhood into adulthood. Lancet Respir Med. 2017;5(3):224–34. doi: S2213-2600(16)30187-4 [pii].
44. Sears MR, Greene JM, Willan AR, et al. A longitudinal, population-based, cohort study of childhood asthma followed to adulthood. N Engl J Med. 2003;349(15):1414–22. https://doi.org/10.1056/NEJMoa022363.
45. Withers AL, Green R. Transition for adolescents and young adults with asthma. Front Pediatr. 2019;7:301. https://doi.org/10.3389/fped.2019.00301.
46. Bergström S, Sundell K, Hedlin G. Adolescents with asthma: consequences of transition from paediatric to adult healthcare. Respir Med. 2010;104(2):180–7. https://doi.org/10.1016/j.rmed.2009.09.021.
47. Scal P, Davern M, Ireland M, Park K. Transition to adulthood: delays and unmet needs among adolescents and young adults with asthma. J Pediatr. 2008;152(4):471–475.e1. https://doi.org/10.1016/j.jpeds.2007.10.004.
48. Odling M, Jonsson M, Janson C, Melen E, Bergstrom A, Kull I. Lost in the transition from pediatric to adult healthcare? Experiences of young adults with severe asthma. J Asthma. 2019;57:1–9. https://doi.org/10.1080/02770903.2019.1640726.
49. Ogawa M, Albrecht D. Adolescence to adulthood: safely transitioning the adolescent with pulmonary arterial hypertension. Adv Pulm Hypertens. 2009;8(4):232–6. https://doi.org/10.2169 3/1933-088X-8.4.232.
50. Barst RJ, Ertel SI, Beghetti M, Ivy DD. Pulmonary arterial hypertension: a comparison between children and adults. Eur Respir J. 2011;37(3):665–77. https://doi.org/10.1183/09031936.00056110.
51. van Loon RL, Roofthooft MT, Delhaas T, et al. Outcome of pediatric patients with pulmonary arterial hypertension in the era of new medical therapies. Am J Cardiol. 2010;106(1):117–24. https://doi.org/10.1016/j.amjcard.2010.02.023.

Part III
Best Practice Recommendations and Transition Outcomes in Specific Pulmonary Conditions

Chapter 7
Providing Care for a Changing CF Population

Katherine Alex Despotes and Jennifer L. Goralski

CF as a Model Disease

Healthcare professionals who provide care for people with cystic fibrosis (CF) have long been at the forefront of advocating for a formal transition process. Despite being almost universally known as a "pediatric" disease, advances in medical care starting in the 1990s have led to an increasing number of people with CF reaching adolescence and young adulthood. The Cystic Fibrosis Foundation (CFF), which accredits CF centers, was an early adopter of the transition model and began to advocate for the development of adult CF care programs in the late 1990s. By the year 2000, the CFF mandated that in order to maintain CFF accreditation, any CF center that provided care to more than 40 patients over the age of 21 must develop and maintain an adult CF program. This was followed by a 2004 consensus guideline on optimal adult CF care [1]. An additional CFF requirement in 2008 subsequently stated all care centers needed to transition 90% of their patients between the ages 18 and 21 to adult care. This allowed for individualization of the timing of transition and special allowances for unique circumstances while ensuring the vast majority of people with CF received age-appropriate care. Coupled with this, to sustain accreditation, centers also had to formalize a structured transition program and organize regular meetings between the pediatric and adult centers.

In response to these recommendations, the number of adult CF care programs grew exponentially. Furthermore, in 2015, adults with CF over the age of 18 outnumbered children with CF for the first time [2]. The CFF has recognized that appropriate training for adult care providers in the nuances of CF is necessary and

K. A. Despotes · J. L. Goralski (✉)
The University of North Carolina at Chapel Hill, Chapel Hill, NC, USA
e-mail: Jennifer_goralski@med.unc.edu

© Springer Nature Switzerland AG 2021   105
C. D. Brown, E. Crowley (eds.), *Transitioning Care from Pediatric to Adult Pulmonology*, Respiratory Medicine,
https://doi.org/10.1007/978-3-030-68688-8_7

has developed programs and funding opportunities to provide additional education and financial support to pulmonologists, endocrinologists, and gastroenterologists who have taken a special interest in the disease.

Change in Disease

Timing of transition for young adults with CF can be particularly onerous, as it coincides with a time of high risk for disease deterioration [2]. Within the anticipated time frame for transition, adolescents are expected to complete high school and enter college or work [3]. They must learn to be independent, both in the realm of their disease management and in their life, in general. Overall, achievement of adult milestones is delayed in adolescents with a chronic health condition compared with age-matched peers [4–6]. In addition, adolescents with a chronic health condition are more likely to suffer from anxiety or depression, and CF is no exception [7]. Mental health disorders frequently lead to issues with medication adherence, which may cause further deterioration in lung health.

The Modulator Era and Changing Needs

The FDA approval of ivacaftor (Kalydeco ©) in 2012 launched a new era in CF treatment. As the first cystic fibrosis transmembrane regulator (CFTR) modulator drug, ivacaftor increased the open-channel probability of the CFTR protein and thus allowed for normalization of sweat chloride levels, improvements in lung function, and enhanced quality of life for the 4% of people with CF who carried the eligible mutations. Indeed, epidemiological studies showed a decline in time to acquisition of new bacteria in the era after the widespread availability of modulators [8]. Ivacaftor was followed by lumacaftor/ivacaftor (Orkambi ©) in 2015 and tezacaftor/ivacaftor (Symdeko ©) in 2017. These pharmacologic agents provided access to modulator therapy for a larger number of CF mutations, though they did not provide the same degree of clinical improvements as was seen with ivacaftor. Nonetheless, they paved the way for the creation of "triple drug therapy" [9–11], a combination of elexacaftor, tezacaftor, and ivacaftor (Trikafta ©), which was granted priority FDA review in 2019 and approved for patients aged 12 and older with at least one copy of Phe508del. With clinical trial data that matches or exceeds the improvements seen in patients eligible for ivacaftor, triple drug therapy offers a robust CFTR corrector/potentiator combination for nearly 90% of patients with CF. Additional modulators are in various stages of clinical trials and portend a time when options for CFTR modulation may be numerous.

With the advent of clinical use of CFTR modulators, the approach to CF transition will almost certainly change in the near future. In the past, pediatric pulmonologists cared for patients with a wide range of lung function deficits, and often, a decision about the appropriate timing of transition was based around clinical health and pulmonary exacerbations. As younger patients become eligible for highly effective CFTR modulators, the overall trajectory of the disease is anticipated to change. Experts expect the majority of people to be managed as a chronic disease, similar to asthma, with fewer flare-ups and generally less severe lung disease. With fewer acute, time-sensitive needs, patients and providers may be able to focus more time on preparing the adolescent to assume responsibility for aspects of chronic disease management.

A generally accepted tenant about transition is that patients should not be transferred to a new adult care team during a period of clinical instability, whether this be during a CF pulmonary exacerbation, treatment for mycobacterial disease, or evaluation for lung transplant. Thus, a number of transitions have been delayed over the years, with patients remaining in pediatric care until their disease stabilizes. Occasionally, patients are rushed into transfer when they reach a period of time where they have temporarily stabilized medically (though perhaps not mentally or socially). With the onset of highly effective modulator treatment, it is anticipated that patients will experience longer periods of clinical stability, thus allowing transition topics to be serially introduced and transfer timing to be appropriately planned.

Best Practices in CF

Despite general acknowledgment of the importance of a planned transition process, significant variation exists in the structure of this process between centers [12–14]. Numerous studies and reviews have attempted to distill the best practices for transition in CF [3, 15–18]. However, most of the recommendations are based on expert opinions and not prospective studies that show improved health outcomes in adults [19]. Part of the challenge is identifying meaningful outcome measures to mark a successful transition [20], particularly in the setting of a severe chronic disease where health may deteriorate in spite of adherence and support. Lanzkron and colleagues [19] advocate for a focus on developing key research questions, recognizing that there are a variety of stakeholders as well as situations (home life, communities, education) that are targeted in transition practices. Recognizing this, the feasibility of randomized controlled clinical trials is in question, so the focus may be better directed to patient registries, quality improvement efforts, and comparative effectiveness research.

Despite this limitation, expert opinion of best practices has repeatedly focused on several topics, including those listed in Table 7.1.

Table 7.1 Best practices in CF transition

Best practice	Examples/comments	References
Ongoing communication between the pediatric and adult care colleagues	Formal transfer meeting Written transfer document Transition clinic	[1, 15, 16, 21]
Use of a validated transition tool to document knowledge and milestones	CF R.I.S.E. Ready, Steady, Go TRAQ STARx	[22–25]
Initiating the process early, potentially from the time of diagnosis	Allows for transition to be a gradual process, permitting the adolescent to develop life skills and disease-specific management	[3, 16]
Supporting parents and caregivers through the process	Unsupported or domineering parents can inhibit the adolescent's ability to achieve independence	[3, 16, 26, 27]
Providing access to a transition navigator who can accompany the patient on their journey through the transition process	May be a nurse, social worker, or transition coordinator	[1, 15]

Need for Multispecialty and Multidisciplinary Involvement in Transition

Although the respiratory system is the primary source of morbidity and mortality, CF is truly a multisystem disease, which must be carefully considered during the transition process. Given the relative rarity of the condition (approximately 30,000 patients in the USA and 70,000 worldwide), optimal CF care and expertise is largely delivered by trained subspecialists at a designated CF center, which is generally considered a medical home for the patients. There are approximately 130 CFF-accredited centers across the country. This could potentially have implications for where a patient may opt to live. Patients who live farther away from the nearest CF center (by choice or out of necessity) may need to rely more on a primary care provider as well as a local pulmonologist, with periodic visits to the CF center. On the other hand, some patients opt to relocate close to a CF center for ready access to experts. In these scenarios, pulmonologists may be viewed by patients as the primary care provider, which can be a challenging dynamic to balance. Pulmonologists should discuss expectations of care delivery frankly with patients and their families. Having a dedicated primary care provider to ensure guidelines for routine adult health and screening are being met may be appropriate, with close communication with the pulmonologist as to how CF impacts these guidelines.

Related to this, while pulmonologists typically play the central role in a patient's care, CF is a multi-organ disease, and the transition process extends to other subspecialties that may also care for the patient. This includes, but is not limited to, providers in gastroenterology, endocrinology, reproductive health, and mental health. The support structures in place for adults with chronic medical conditions can vary significantly from supports available to children with medical conditions. This includes navigating insurance coverage and advocating for appropriate accommodations in education and in the workforce.

Pulmonary

Adolescence is a particularly vulnerable period in the disease course for patients with CF [28]. Pulmonary function decline is most rapid during adolescence and early adulthood, during the same time frame as the typical transition period [2, 29]. Challenges with compliance (in part related to treatment burden, declining parental supervision, and increasing independence) in this age group have been thought to contribute to the decline in lung function during this period [30–32]. Increased exacerbation frequency has also been noted as a contributing factor to this accelerated loss of lung function [33]. Worse nutritional status, as discussed below, has also been tied to declining lung function.

Lung transplantation remains an important avenue of treatment for individuals with advanced CF lung disease. In addition to the transition from pediatric to adult care, some patients will require additional coordination of care between their CF center and a transplant center. Early referral is important for patients and families to be fully educated about the medical, psychosocial, and financial aspects of transplant, should the need arise in the future [34].

Gastroenterology

People with CF have an increased prevalence of pre-cancerous adenomatous polyps [35] and colon cancers [36, 37]. Updated colorectal cancer screening recommendations, endorsed by the CF Foundation, were outlined in 2017, including the recommendation to begin screening at 40 years old rather than the age of 50 recommended for the general population [38]. Patients should undergo repeat screening every 5 years (or more frequently, depending on colonoscopy findings) [38]. People with CF who have undergone solid organ transplantation should start screening at age 30 as a result of the increased risk of colon cancer related to immunosuppression [38].

As part of efforts to improve the transition from pediatric to adult care, the CF Foundation has made a significant investment in the training of adult subspecialty providers, including the DIGEST program to foster development of gastroenterology subspecialists who have an interest in caring for people with CF. Ideally, people with CF should be cared for by a gastroenterologist who is knowledgeable about CF and familiar with the CF-specific screening guidelines [38]. At a minimum, there is a need for coordination with the patient's CF provider and the gastroenterologist, as many CF centers do not have an adult gastroenterologist with specific training in CF manifestations. It is important for gastroenterologists to understand that patients with CF often require more intensive bowel prep for screening colonoscopy [39]. The sedation and procedural risks are also higher during colonoscopy for patients with CF compared with the general population, dependent on the degree of lung function impairment [38].

Nutrition plays an integral role in lung function and overall health in people with CF, with low body weight correlating with increased mortality and decreased lung function [40, 41]. Current recommendations for patients ages 2–20 include maintaining a BMI of ≥50th percentile [42]. Adult patients with CF should strive for BMI of >22 kg/m² for women and >23 kg/m² for men [42]. CF nutritionists integrated into the multidisciplinary CF care team are key in monitoring weight and growth and guiding nutrition therapy.

Endocrinology

CF-related diabetes (CFRD) also increases in incidence with age [43, 44]. CFRD is a distinctive clinical entity from Type 1 diabetes mellitus (DM) and Type 2 DM [45]. Patients with pancreatic insufficiency are at highest risk of developing CFRD, and many are identified with abnormal glucose tolerance in adolescence, with the diagnosis of CFRD occurring during this pivotal transition period from pediatric to adult care [43]. Thus, regular screening starting at age 10 is crucial for identification of patients at risk for CFRD, and early diabetes education should occur as CFRD also has significant treatment burden [43, 46]. Furthermore, diagnosing and monitoring CFRD is challenging because, in CF, hemoglobin A1c is not always well correlated to blood sugar levels [45, 47]. Data for treating CFRD is limited to using insulin, which is needed not only to manage hyperglycemia but also to ensure utilization of caloric intake to support nutritional status and lung function [45]. There is currently no role for the use of oral hypoglycemic agents in CFRD. The goals for treatment during the transition period include maintaining blood glucose control and preserving pulmonary function [43]. Ideally patients should see a CF endocrinologist quarterly, in conjunction with their pulmonologist and multidisciplinary team.

Bone health is impacted by several factors in CF (malnutrition, vitamin D and calcium deficiency, steroid exposure, and inflammation, among others) [48]. Prevalence of osteopenia and osteoporosis have risen with the increased longevity of people with CF [49], and closer attention to bone health earlier in childhood and adolescence may prevent subsequent morbidity in adulthood. In 2005, the CF Foundation issued recommendations related to bone density screening. Current recommendations include initiation of dual-energy X-ray absorptiometry (DXA) as early as age 8 if patients weigh <90% ideal body weight, if decreased lung function with FEV1 < 50% predicted, if on prolonged courses of steroids, or if there is a history of delayed puberty or history of fractures [48]. Adult care providers should be aware to start screening all people with CF at age 18, if not previously screened

[49]. Despite recommendations for screening, there is significant complexity in interpreting DXA results for people with CF [48]. Treatment recommendations include improving nutritional status, and ensuring adequate vitamin D, calcium, and vitamin K supplementation, along with weight bearing exercise and adequate sunlight exposure. Bisphosphonates have demonstrated benefit in individuals with a Z-score of less than −2. Providers should minimize steroid use whenever possible [48].

Given the unique features of managing CFRD and other endocrine disorders associated with CF (osteopenia and osteoporosis, reproductive health, etc.), the ENVISION program sponsored by the CFF offers support and training to endocrinology subspecialists who embark on specific training to care for people with CF.

Reproductive Health

Reproductive health education is often overlooked by physicians given the numerous other health priorities [50, 51]. People with CF have indicated that they would like their physician to discuss infertility, pregnancy planning, and pregnancy prevention with them [50, 52, 53]. Particularly for men, of whom >95% cannot father a child naturally, education about the congenital absence of the vas deferens needs to be undertaken as soon as developmentally appropriate, along with the explicit statement that this infertility does not protect against sexually transmitted infection (STI) transmission. These discussions, including STI prevention and other aspects of sexual health, should begin in adolescence, similar to young adults without a chronic disease [50, 51]. Adult care providers will need to continue these conversations following the transition from pediatric care, as patients' reproductive goals may shift from pregnancy prevention to desiring conception [52]. Women should receive counseling on the risks of pregnancy depending on their pulmonary function, as well as risks to the fetus, particularly in the era of CFTR modulation, where there is limited understanding of the effects of modulators on a developing fetus [52, 53]. It should be noted that the CFF has convened a working group on women's health initiatives, which will explore the best way to assess safety of modulator therapy during pregnancy/lactation. All patients desiring conception should be offered genetic counseling [52] and genetic testing of the unaffected partner. Pregnancy in CF should be ideally managed at a center with a close relationship between the CF team and the obstetrician [52, 53].

Mental Health

The CFF has emphasized the need for routine screening for anxiety and depression and the importance of treatment of mental health conditions [54]. Rates of depression and anxiety increase during adolescence for many patients with CF and continue to rise in adulthood [54]. If untreated, anxiety and depression may hinder the transition process, just as comorbid mental health issues impact adherence with treatments and healthcare utilization [19, 54]. Psychological interventions such as cognitive behavioral therapy are encouraged, with the addition of pharmacological therapy if symptoms are moderate to severe. Medication management should ideally be carried out in conjunction with a mental health provider and with special attention to patients' other CF medications and conditions. Medication dose reductions as well as increases (depending on absorption) may be required [54].

Education and the Workforce

Due to longer life expectancy, more people with CF are attending college and pursuing employment [19]. According to the CFF Adult Clinical Care guidelines, providers should engage patients in discussion about career planning and higher education and help advise on the implications of CF on their education and jobs [1]. Patients should be informed of their rights under the Americans with Disabilities Act (ADA), which includes being entitled to accommodations such as additional sick time or an adjusted work schedule. Potential employers cannot ask if an individual has a medical condition or disability during the application process; however, the individual may decide to disclose their diagnosis once securing a position. The CF center can be useful in providing accurate information about the diagnosis to the employer in these situations.

Similarly, individuals who are starting college should be informed of their rights under the ADA. The CF center may need to corroborate information about the patient's medical condition and need for accommodations. Patients who relocate to attend college should investigate access to care, including local CF centers near their institution [1].

One aspect of care that is very uncertain is how CFTR modulators will impact access to higher education and career selection. Patients who are healthier throughout childhood and adolescence may choose to pursue more challenging careers or additional education. Previously, these pathways may have been considered less worthwhile to those with a markedly limited lifespan.

The long-term impact of CFTR modulators on people with CF in the workforce and eligibility for disability also remains to be seen. Lack of insurance has been associated with less frequent use of routine care in people with CF [55]. Under the Affordable Care Act (ACA) in 2010, insurance coverage was expanded to allow dependent children ages 19–25 to remain on their parents' insurance. However, initial studies have not shown an increase in insurance coverage or utilization of routine care in people with CF in this age group [56]. This is likely explained by a higher percentage of adults with CF already maintaining health insurance compared to age-matched adults in the general population. Even after the age of 25, people with CF may or may not be able to sustain full-time employment with benefits, due to the intense and time-consuming daily treatments required. Social workers and the COMPASS program through the CFF can help patients navigate the multiple options available for coverage.

Training Adult Care Providers

The transition from pediatric care to adult care is challenging but necessary as patients age and their care needs change [19]. In accordance with the joint statement put forth by the AAP, ACP, and AAFP in 2011 and updated in 2018, pediatric and adult providers will share in the responsibility for healthcare transitions [57]. In the past, adult and pediatric providers reported that they were not comfortable with guiding patients through transitions [58], but as more patients age into adulthood, this will become an increasingly necessary part of training physicians and other medical disciplines. In general, trainees in combined programs (Internal Medicine/Pediatrics) had the highest levels of reported confidence in transition care, and this exposure to the age range of adolescents and young adults can be mimicked through specific transition curricula in residency and fellowship [57, 59, 60].

Conclusion

Cystic fibrosis, long considered a "pediatric disease," has benefited from improved nutrition management, eradication of pathogens, and modulators of CFTR, which have extended the lifespan of people living with this disease. Best practices of transition in CF will serve as a model for other disease processes that bridge the lifespan of patients.

References

1. Yankaskas JR, Marshall BC, Sufian B, Simon RH, Rodman D. Cystic fibrosis adult care: consensus conference report. Chest. 2004;125(1 Suppl):1s–39s.
2. 2015 Annual Data Report [Internet]. 2015. Available from: https://www.cff.org/Our-Research/CF-Patient-Registry/2015-Patient-Registry-Annual-Data-Report.pdf.
3. Goralski JL, Nasr SZ, Uluer A. Overcoming barriers to a successful transition from pediatric to adult care. Pediatr Pulmonol. 2017;52(S48):S52–60.
4. Pfeffer PE, Pfeffer JM, Hodson ME. The psychosocial and psychiatric side of cystic fibrosis in adolescents and adults. J Cyst Fibros. 2003;2(2):61–8.
5. Stam H, Hartman EE, Deurloo JA, Groothoff J, Grootenhuis MA. Young adult patients with a history of pediatric disease: impact on course of life and transition into adulthood. J Adolesc Health. 2006;39(1):4–13.
6. Congleton J, Hodson ME, Duncan-Skingle F. Quality of life in adults with cystic fibrosis. Thorax. 1996;51(9):936–40.

7. Besier T, Born A, Henrich G, Hinz A, Quittner AL, Goldbeck L. Anxiety, depression, and life satisfaction in parents caring for children with cystic fibrosis. Pediatr Pulmonol. 2011;46(7):672–82.
8. Singh SB, McLearn-Montz AJ, Milavetz F, Gates LK, Fox C, Murry LT, et al. Pathogen acquisition in patients with cystic fibrosis receiving ivacaftor or lumacaftor/ivacaftor. Pediatr Pulmonol. 2019;54(8):1200–8.
9. Davies JC, Moskowitz SM, Brown C, Horsley A, Mall MA, McKone EF, et al. VX-659-Tezacaftor-ivacaftor in patients with cystic fibrosis and one or two Phe508del alleles. N Engl J Med. 2018;379(17):1599–611.
10. Heijerman HGM, McKone EF, Downey DG, Van Braeckel E, Rowe SM, Tullis E, et al. Efficacy and safety of the elexacaftor plus tezacaftor plus ivacaftor combination regimen in people with cystic fibrosis homozygous for the F508del mutation: a double-blind, randomised, phase 3 trial. Lancet (London, England). 2019;394(10212):1940–8.
11. Middleton PG, Mall MA, Drevinek P, Lands LC, McKone EF, Polineni D, et al. Elexacaftor-Tezacaftor-Ivacaftor for cystic fibrosis with a single Phe508del allele. N Engl J Med. 2019;381(19):1809–19.
12. Tuchman L, Schwartz M. Health outcomes associated with transition from pediatric to adult cystic fibrosis care. Pediatrics. 2013;132(5):847–53.
13. Nasr SZ, Campbell C, Howatt W. Transition program from pediatric to adult care for cystic fibrosis patients. J Adolesc Health. 1992;13(8):682–5.
14. Askew K, Bamford J, Hudson N, Moratelli J, Miller R, Anderson A, et al. Current characteristics, challenges and coping strategies of young people with cystic fibrosis as they transition to adulthood. Clin Med (Lond). 2017;17(2):121–5.
15. Okumura MJ, Kleinhenz ME. Cystic fibrosis transitions of care: lessons learned and future directions for cystic fibrosis. Clin Chest Med. 2016;37(1):119–26.
16. West NE, Mogayzel PJ Jr. Transitions in health care: what can we learn from our experience with cystic fibrosis. Pediatr Clin N Am. 2016;63(5):887–97.
17. Flume PA. Smoothing the transition from pediatric to adult care: lessons learned. Curr Opin Pulm Med. 2009;15(6):611–4.
18. Campbell F, Biggs K, Aldiss SK, O'Neill PM, Clowes M, McDonagh J, et al. Transition of care for adolescents from paediatric services to adult health services. Cochrane Database Syst Rev. 2016;4:CD009794.
19. Lanzkron S, Sawicki GS, Hassell KL, Konstan MW, Liem RI, McColley SA. Transition to adulthood and adult health care for patients with sickle cell disease or cystic fibrosis: current practices and research priorities. J Clin Transl Sci. 2018;2(5):334–42.
20. Fair C, Cuttance J, Sharma N, Maslow G, Wiener L, Betz C, et al. International and interdisciplinary identification of health care transition outcomes. JAMA Pediatr. 2016;170(3):205–11.
21. Dugueperoux I, Tamalet A, Sermet-Gaudelus I, Le Bourgeois M, Gerardin M, Desmazes-Dufeu N, et al. Clinical changes of patients with cystic fibrosis during transition from pediatric to adult care. J Adolesc Health. 2008;43(5):459–65.
22. Baker AM, Riekert KA, Sawicki GS, Eakin MN. CF RISE: implementing a clinic-based transition program. Pediatr Allergy Immunol Pulmonol. 2015;28(4):250–4.
23. Nagra A, McGinnity PM, Davis N, Salmon AP. Implementing transition: ready steady go. Arch Dis Child Educ Pract Ed. 2015;100(6):313–20.
24. Sawicki GS, Lukens-Bull K, Yin X, Demars N, Huang IC, Livingood W, et al. Measuring the transition readiness of youth with special healthcare needs: validation of the TRAQ – Transition Readiness Assessment Questionnaire. J Pediatr Psychol. 2011;36(2):160–71.
25. Ferris M, Cohen S, Haberman C, Javalkar K, Massengill S, Mahan JD, et al. Self-management and transition readiness assessment: development, reliability, and factor structure of the STARx questionnaire. J Pediatr Nurs. 2015;30(5):691–9.
26. Iles N, Lowton K. What is the perceived nature of parental care and support for young people with cystic fibrosis as they enter adult health services? Health Soc Care Community. 2010;18(1):21–9.

27. Huang JS, Gottschalk M, Pian M, Dillon L, Barajas D, Bartholomew LK. Transition to adult care: systematic assessment of adolescents with chronic illnesses and their medical teams. J Pediatr. 2011;159(6):994–8 e2.
28. Bowmer G, Sowerby C, Duff A. Transition and transfer of young people with cystic fibrosis to adult care. Nurs Child Young People. 2018;30(5):34–9.
29. Vandenbranden SL, McMullen A, Schechter MS, Pasta DJ, Michaelis RL, Konstan MW, et al. Lung function decline from adolescence to young adulthood in cystic fibrosis. Pediatr Pulmonol. 2012;47(2):135–43.
30. Bishay LC, Sawicki GS. Strategies to optimize treatment adherence in adolescent patients with cystic fibrosis. Adolesc Health Med Ther. 2016;7:117–24.
31. Zemanick ET, Harris JK, Conway S, Konstan MW, Marshall B, Quittner AL, et al. Measuring and improving respiratory outcomes in cystic fibrosis lung disease: opportunities and challenges to therapy. J Cyst Fibros. 2010;9(1):1–16.
32. George M, Rand-Giovannetti D, Eakin MN, Borrelli B, Zettler M, Riekert KA. Perceptions of barriers and facilitators: self-management decisions by older adolescents and adults with CF. J Cyst Fibros. 2010;9(6):425–32.
33. Konstan MW, Morgan WJ, Butler SM, Pasta DJ, Craib ML, Silva SJ, et al. Risk factors for rate of decline in forced expiratory volume in one second in children and adolescents with cystic fibrosis. J Pediatr. 2007;151(2):134–9, 9 e1.
34. Ramos KJ, Smith PJ, McKone EF, Pilewski JM, Lucy A, Hempstead SE, et al. Lung transplant referral for individuals with cystic fibrosis: Cystic Fibrosis Foundation consensus guidelines. J Cyst Fibros. 2019;18(3):321–33.
35. Hegagi M, Aaron SD, James P, Goel R, Chatterjee A. Increased prevalence of colonic adenomas in patients with cystic fibrosis. J Cyst Fibros. 2017;16(6):759–62.
36. Neglia JP, FitzSimmons SC, Maisonneuve P, Schoni MH, Schoni-Affolter F, Corey M, et al. The risk of cancer among patients with cystic fibrosis. Cystic Fibrosis and Cancer Study Group. N Engl J Med. 1995;332(8):494–9.
37. Maisonneuve P, Marshall BC, Knapp EA, Lowenfels AB. Cancer risk in cystic fibrosis: a 20-year nationwide study from the United States. J Natl Cancer Inst. 2013;105(2):122–9.
38. Hadjiliadis D, Khoruts A, Zauber AG, Hempstead SE, Maisonneuve P, Lowenfels AB, et al. Cystic fibrosis colorectal cancer screening consensus recommendations. Gastroenterology. 2018;154(3):736–45. e14
39. Matson AG, Bunting JP, Kaul A, Smith DJ, Stonestreet J, Herd K, et al. A non-randomised single centre cohort study, comparing standard and modified bowel preparations, in adults with cystic fibrosis requiring colonoscopy. BMC Gastroenterol. 2019;19(1):89.
40. Salvatore D, Buzzetti R, Mastella G. Update of literature from cystic fibrosis registries 2012-2015. Part 6: epidemiology, nutrition and complications. Pediatr Pulmonol. 2017;52(3):390–8.
41. Forrester DL, Knox AJ, Smyth AR, Fogarty AW. Measures of body habitus are associated with lung function in adults with cystic fibrosis: a population-based study. J Cyst Fibros. 2013;12(3):284–9.
42. Stallings VA, Stark LJ, Robinson KA, Feranchak AP, Quinton H, Clinical Practice Guidelines on G, et al. Evidence-based practice recommendations for nutrition-related management of children and adults with cystic fibrosis and pancreatic insufficiency: results of a systematic review. J Am Diet Assoc. 2008;108(5):832–9.
43. Middleton PG, Matson AG, Robinson PD, Jane Holmes-Walker D, Katz T, Hameed S. Cystic fibrosis related diabetes: potential pitfalls in the transition from paediatric to adult care. Paediatr Respir Rev. 2014;15(3):281–4.
44. Chamnan P, Shine BS, Haworth CS, Bilton D, Adler AI. Diabetes as a determinant of mortality in cystic fibrosis. Diabetes Care. 2010;33(2):311–6.
45. Konrad K, Scheuing N, Badenhoop K, Borkenstein MH, Gohlke B, Schofl C, et al. Cystic fibrosis-related diabetes compared with type 1 and type 2 diabetes in adults. Diabetes Metab Res Rev. 2013;29(7):568–75.

46. Moran A, Brunzell C, Cohen RC, Katz M, Marshall BC, Onady G, et al. Clinical care guidelines for cystic fibrosis-related diabetes: a position statement of the American Diabetes Association and a clinical practice guideline of the Cystic Fibrosis Foundation, endorsed by the Pediatric Endocrine Society. Diabetes Care. 2010;33(12):2697–708.
47. Godbout A, Hammana I, Potvin S, Mainville D, Rakel A, Berthiaume Y, et al. No relationship between mean plasma glucose and glycated haemoglobin in patients with cystic fibrosis-related diabetes. Diabetes Metab. 2008;34(6 Pt 1):568–73.
48. Aris RM, Merkel PA, Bachrach LK, Borowitz DS, Boyle MP, Elkin SL, et al. Guide to bone health and disease in cystic fibrosis. J Clin Endocrinol Metab. 2005;90(3):1888–96.
49. Stalvey MS, Clines GA. Cystic fibrosis-related bone disease: insights into a growing problem. Curr Opin Endocrinol Diabetes Obes. 2013;20(6):547–52.
50. Sawyer SM, Farrant B, Cerritelli B, Wilson J. A survey of sexual and reproductive health in men with cystic fibrosis: new challenges for adolescent and adult services. Thorax. 2005;60(4):326–30.
51. Withers AL. Management issues for adolescents with cystic fibrosis. Pulm Med. 2012;2012:134132.
52. Lyon A, Bilton D. Fertility issues in cystic fibrosis. Paediatr Respir Rev. 2002;3(3):236–40.
53. Roberts S, Green P. The sexual health of adolescents with cystic fibrosis. J R Soc Med. 2005;98 Suppl 45:7–16.
54. Quittner AL, Abbott J, Georgiopoulos AM, Goldbeck L, Smith B, Hempstead SE, et al. International Committee on Mental Health in Cystic Fibrosis: Cystic Fibrosis Foundation and European Cystic Fibrosis Society consensus statements for screening and treating depression and anxiety. Thorax. 2016;71(1):26–34.
55. Li SS, Hayes D Jr, Tobias JD, Morgan WJ, Tumin D. Health insurance and use of recommended routine care in adults with cystic fibrosis. Clin Respir J. 2018;12(5):1981–8.
56. Tumin D, Li SS, Kopp BT, Kirkby SE, Tobias JD, Morgan WJ, et al. The effect of the affordable care act dependent coverage provision on patients with cystic fibrosis. Pediatr Pulmonol. 2017;52(4):458–66.
57. White PH, Cooley WC, Transitions Clinical Report Authoring Group, American Academy of Pediatrics, American Academy of Family Physicians, American College of Physicians. Supporting the health care transition from adolescence to adulthood in the medical home. Pediatrics. 2018;142(5):e20182587. https://doi.org/10.1542/peds.2018–2587. Epub 2018 Oct 22. Erratum in: Pediatrics. 2019;143(2): PMID: 30348754.
58. Okumura MJ, Heisler M, Davis MM, Cabana MD, Demonner S, Kerr EA. Comfort of general internists and general pediatricians in providing care for young adults with chronic illnesses of childhood. J Gen Intern Med. 2008;23(10):1621–7.
59. Patel MS, O'Hare K. Residency training in transition of youth with childhood-onset chronic disease. Pediatrics. 2010;126 Suppl 3:S190–3.
60. Sadun RE, Chung RJ, Pollock MD, Maslow GR. Lost in transition: resident and fellow training and experience caring for young adults with chronic conditions in a large United States' academic medical center. Med Educ Online. 2019;24(1):1605783.

Chapter 8
Transition Care for Adolescents and Young Adults with Neuromuscular Disease and Chronic Pulmonary Care Needs

Kathleen S. Irby and Jeanette P. Brown

Case JW is a 19-year-old woman with a history of spinal muscular atrophy (SMA) type II. Her symptoms started at 12 months old, when she had difficulty in sitting without support. She has scoliosis and chest wall deformities requiring spinal fusion. She was able to crawl but never was able to walk unaided. She uses a motorized wheelchair for mobility. She was treated as a child at a tertiary children's hospital. She was found to have respiratory muscle weakness with a forced vital capacity (FVC) of 0.51 L, 26% predicted, and has been using nocturnal bi-level positive pressure ventilation for support. She uses a mechanical insufflator/exsufflator device for cough assistance. She will now be attending college and she presents to the adult pulmonary clinic to establish care and long-term follow-up. She has to deal with changing insurance and moving to a new state, as well as getting to know a new doctor and clinic.

Introduction

Chronic neuromuscular respiratory failure is a consequence of a number of conditions that first present in childhood, such as myotonic dystrophy and spinal muscular atrophy (SMA). Many of these patients are treated at pediatric hospital specialty clinics, such as Shriners Hospitals or Muscular Dystrophy Association (MDA) clinics, although some patients may be followed by individual pediatric providers

K. S. Irby
Internal Medicine-Pediatrics, University of Utah, Salt Lake City, UT, USA

J. P. Brown (✉)
Internal Medicine Division of Pulmonary, Critical Care & Occupational Pulmonary, University of Utah, Salt Lake City, UT, USA
e-mail: Jeanette.Brown@hsc.utah.edu

© Springer Nature Switzerland AG 2021
C. D. Brown, E. Crowley (eds.), *Transitioning Care from Pediatric to Adult Pulmonology*, Respiratory Medicine,
https://doi.org/10.1007/978-3-030-68688-8_8

(subspecialty and primary care). Multidisciplinary clinics have provided these children comprehensive care including social work, dieticians, physiatrists, neurologists, pulmonologists, and others. This care has extended the life span for these conditions and many patients are now living into adulthood [8]. Though epidemiological data is quite limited for most neuromuscular diseases, incidence of SMA is cited at 1 per 6,000–10,000 live births with prevalence of 1–2 per 100,000 persons. Duchenne and Becker muscular dystrophies come to an incidence of 1 per 3500–5000 male births, meaning approximately 400–600 affected males born in the USA annually [12, 13, 15, 21, 24]. The frequencies of many conditions, including rare diseases, are often unknown as there are no active registries.

Advancements in mechanical ventilators and mechanical insufflation/exsufflation devices over the last 30 plus years have made them smaller and easier to use. These advances have facilitated the transfer of care for children with chronic neuromuscular respiratory failure to the home environment instead of long-term residency in medical institutions [27]. Improvements in mask technology and mouthpiece ventilation have allowed patients to avoid tracheostomy as well [3]. Patients with Duchenne muscular dystrophy (DMD) and SMA are now living longer. There is drastic variation on life expectancy across the spectrum of clinical manifestations in these conditions. Over the past couple of decades, patients with DMD experienced an increase in life expectancy of more than 10 years, with now routinely living into third decade of life [25]. People with SMA are experiencing an unprecedented and undefined expansion of life expectancy with new disease-modifying agents. With this increased survival, the need for organized transition from pediatric to adult providers has become more important [2, 7, 16, 31].

There are a number of transitions in the process of going from pediatric to adult pulmonary care for these patients who may be device-dependent. The structure of pulmonary training in the USA also plays a role in the transition as well. Providers are typically trained in pediatrics or internal medicine first before subspecialization, meaning that there are not classically pulmonologists cross-trained in adult and pediatric medicine. This requires patients to transition from one practice environment to the other with respect to respiratory management. Exact timing has been debated for this transfer of care. Challenges include having adult providers that are familiar with the underlying neuromuscular conditions and willing to engage with these complex patients. Pediatric tertiary clinics also typically have more support staff and services, such as social work, that are often lacking in standard adult pulmonary clinics. Replacing these services on the adult side of the transition is challenging and can leave patients and caregivers without as many resources.

Coordinating a planned transition has been proposed by a number of organizations. The Got Transition website is a collaborative project designed to help guide the process for both pediatric and adult providers. It has many helpful resources, but is not specific for subspecialties. In this chapter, we will discuss patient-centered models that are specific to pediatric to adult transition for patients who are ventilator-dependent due to chronic neuromuscular respiratory failure.

Logistics

As JW is heading off to college, she certainly has medical factors to consider, but there are also several logistical issues that will impact her next steps. She needs to find providers to help adjust her respiratory support and medications, but she also needs to find housing that can accommodate her devices and figure out transportation on campus. The logistical challenges faced by adolescents and young adults (AYA) transitioning with chronic disease, such as MD, are as important, arguably more so, than the medical aspects of their transition and require attention and support through the process. Patients' quality of life and reaching maximal functional independence can benefit greatly from involvement of a multidisciplinary support team familiar with community resources and the issues common in this population.

Ideally, for these patients, social workers (SW) or case managers familiar with local resources and policy are an integral part of clinical care. If this is not feasible for a clinic, these providers should be made as available as possible, and regularly updated lists of community organizations should be easily accessible to patients and families. Care managers and social workers who are well informed of community resources for people with neuromuscular disorders (NMDs) can provide invaluable insight and assistance in these situations and ideally should be a central part of the multidisciplinary teams caring for children and adults.

One of the major transitions that people with NMD experience is moving to independent housing or, alternatively, navigating the transition into a young adult in the family home. This change may be prompted by starting higher education, entering the workforce or a vocational program, or aging out of the public school system. For those with significant cognitive delay or severe physical impairment, living independently may not be a realistic option [4]. Others are best served by transitioning to a group home or transitional/supportive environment separate from the family home. Many will be able to transition to independent housing, which comes with its own unique challenges and rewards. It is extremely important to ascertain the wishes, fears, and goals of patients and families when addressing changes to the living environment [18]. Many patients and families find attaining physical independence to be a vital aspect of the adult experience, and they place great value in facing any challenges necessary to allow for independent living. Others may not find this to be their most important goal and would prefer to focus their energy on other areas of achievement while remaining in the family home. Providers should aim to focus encouragement, support, and resources on what is most important to the patient, which may not necessarily fit with traditional models defining what it means to be a high-functioning adult [30].

Aging into young adulthood in the same living environment still requires adjustment by the patient and family with regard to roles in the home, independence and autonomy in engaging in social time and self-care, and social and romantic relationships as age appropriate. Even more relevant than objective age is the patient's cognitive and emotional maturity, which does not match chronological age for many patients with chronic illness. These young adults may also be potentially taking more of a role in the financial and chore support of the household. Even if the patient's physical location is not independent, they can still progress in functional and social independence. This is another area in which adequate counseling and social work support can be of great value to patients and families. Many children grow up reliant on their caregivers for much more (and for much longer) than the average child; self-care issues such as toileting, bathing, medication regimens, self-cathing, wound care, and obtaining nutrition (whether orally or via enteral support) are complex aspects of care in a developing adolescent and warrant dedicated attention from providers to ensure that patients take on as much autonomy as safely possible. It is also worthy of time and care as some patients may need more, rather than less, assistance as they age and experience disease progression.

Patients and families not only need to navigate the in-home social changes during this time, but also the logistical support of a growing and maturing child in the home. Depending on the state of residence, there are varying levels of support available for young adults needing environmental modification, assistive devices, and support and recreational groups. The amount of public financial support for patients with NMD also varies by state [30]. Many AYA must navigate a profound change in resources as they age out of school-centered supports [23]. Under the Individuals with Disabilities Education Act of 1975, students must be provided with free, appropriate public education in the least restrictive environment possible. These services begin with early intervention at ages 0–2 years and special education services ages 3–21 years. Also under this law, students must have a personal transition plan by 16 years of age and work toward developing functional skills [33]. Though many students rely heavily on the educational environment and feel the loss of leaving high school, these transition plans and skills can be very useful in moving into the vocational training realm, as well as into various other levels of community engagement, education, and employment.

The path to independent living in the community and/or utilizing vocational training can be complex and confusing. Resources vary greatly between communities, requiring more support from social work and community organizations to identify housing options. On an individual basis, factors such as accommodations for degree of disability (elevators, ADA-friendly countertops and bathrooms, etc.) and adequate accommodations for devices (electrical plugs, physical space in bedrooms and bathrooms, etc.) need to be addressed. It is also important to find an environment appropriate for the person's level of social and psychological abilities and comfort. There are numerous community, federal, state, and local government programs that can facilitate services, but knowing the specifics of the patient's local area is key. Some potentially helpful programs include Assistive Technology Resource Centers, the local Department of Health and Human Services (which can be helpful in identifying local resources, completing registrations, and getting on wait lists), and local branches of disability services. Home caregivers can be very helpful, with payment through community groups, insurance, or private pay.

Vocational training is a particularly valuable opportunity for many people with chronic conditions, as many are excellent candidates for adapted training and work environments despite deficits in academic, social, and physical functioning [26]. If joining the traditional workforce, patients should be encouraged to find employment that fulfills their interests and needs while balancing the needs of their medical conditions (transportation, physicality of the job, time needed for appointments and treatments, etc.). They should be aware of legal protections for people with disabilities and familiarize themselves with available recourse if being treated unfairly. The Rehabilitation Act of 1973 initiated the movement of equal rights and protections for people with disabilities and has been followed by several other legal statutes that support this population. Under this Act, organizations receiving federal money or that are federal programs cannot discriminate on the basis of disability [36]. The Americans with Disabilities Act of 1990 was a huge step forward for this population, mandating modifications to buildings and public spaces to make them accessible to all and supporting services for those with vision or hearing impairment [1]. The following resources may be a helpful place to start for questions and support:

- American Civil Liberties Union Disability Rights Program, www.aclu.org/disability
- Disability.gov
- https://www.ada.gov/cguide.htm

Transportation also poses unique challenges. If feasible and desired, providers can assist in facilitating acquiring a driver's license and vehicle. Again, working with social work and community resources to find best solutions for transportation needs is an important part of transition planning. Several forms of public transportation may suffice in areas with adequate routes and schedules. Smaller programs for individuals with specific needs may be accessible through community organizations. Much of the discussion about transportation goals (license, etc.) and solving problems, like how to get to school, work, and social activities, should be ongoing through the early years of the transition process but may need refinement as young adults gain more independence and autonomy.

People seeking traditional higher education may benefit from a more directed line of next steps involving student housing or other housing options based through their institution, with clearly designated staff to help students navigate institution-sponsored housing options. When entering higher education, any student (and especially those with any physical or educational disabilities) is required to take over the role of being their own advocate. While most settings in the pediatric world allow for a caregiver or provider to intervene on behalf of the patient, higher education requires a greater degree of autonomy and self-reliance. Students need to have a clear understanding of their role in this arena and acquire the self-help tools they need to reach out to school officials to register their disability and engage in sufficient support services. Many students make the mistake of trying to adapt on their own to the new environment and end up frustrated with a wasted semester before they engage with the school to obtain appropriate accommodations. For example, students with audio or visual disabilities may benefit from extra time for exams, note writing services, or vision/hearing devices during lectures. Limitations with fine motor skills may require adaptations to use computers or completing written assignments or exams. Students dependent on a wheelchair may need assistance with building a schedule that coincides with wheelchair-accessible bus routes, ADA-accessible classrooms and elevators, and adequate time between classes to get across campus safely and complete any medication or treatment regimens. Similarly, student housing considerations will need to include ADA-accessible facilities and sufficient space and plug-ins, etc., for equipment. Below are some potentially help-ful sources of information:

- FERPA, www2.ed.gov, regarding privacy of student records
- IDEA, https://sites.ed.gov/idea/

So how does JW begin to tackle these challenges to reach her goals? Thankfully, in her situation, she has benefitted from strong support from her family and clinic providers through her adolescence. She has not learned to drive and is not inter-ested in pursuing that goal. She has been able to use public transportation in her home city but is concerned that the bus routes in her new college town may not fit her class schedule. She is also concerned that the usual freshman dorms do not have adequate elevator access or bathroom and dorm room adaptations that will allow her to live with her peers. She is also concerned about moving between classes fast enough and completing exams in the regularly allotted time. In high school, she had an Individualized Education Plan (IEP) that accommodated her educational experience to allow her the best chance of success. Without that, she is nervous about not succeeding in her first year. Luckily, her college has an office that actively supports students with disabilities. Using the self-help skills she developed during her transition process, she reaches out to the office well before the start of the semester. This office is able to help her secure student housing in a different building that meets her needs and has the space for a personal caregiver to help her with treatments and care a couple of times per week. She arranges a class schedule that has adequate time to support her mobility needs and intentional breaks to allow her to perform her medical treatments and take medications. She articulates what accommodations she needs from her professors ahead of time, with letters of support as needed from her medical providers. Finally, JW finds a local organization that can give her rides to/from clinic appointments and the gro-cery store. Her parents are able to pick her up for school breaks and the occasional weekend. Clearly, the process of starting college is much more complex for these patients. They likely have the same fears and worries as typical new students, with the addition of fears and worries related to their disease process. Extra support and preparation can go a long way in setting our patients up for success as they navi-gate the adult world.

Insurance coverage continues to be a critical factor in determining the location, providers, and the extent of resources available to all patients in the USA, with particular importance to patients with chronic conditions and high levels of medical need. As patients enter adolescence, it is critical that providers incorporate regular and detailed discussions about future insurance coverage into appointments and transition planning. Patients have several potential sources of insurance. Under the Affordable Care Act (ACA), many patients can remain on their parents' insurance policy until age 26. There are potential state-by-state continuations of coverage if the dependent is unable to self-support. ACA legislation also eliminated exclusions for pre-existing conditions and caps on lifetime coverage. Also facilitated under the ACA, personal policies can be found on the Healthcare Exchange [44]. Many patients with a NMD qualify for benefits under Supplemental Security Income (SSI) and Social Security Disability Insurance (SSDI), which correlates with qualifying for Medicaid coverage. In many states, qualifying for SSI automatically qualifies for Medicaid. In 11 states, an additional application is required. Patients can potentially get Medicaid in states that expanded under ACA if they do not qualify for SSI. Patients enrolled in higher education may have access to private insurance through their institution. Discussions about plans for insurance coverage as patients age into adulthood should begin early in the transition process and involve patients, parents, and the care team with the goal of avoiding any lapses in care. As patients are transitioning to their adult care teams, attention should be given to availability of appropriate in-network providers wherever patients will be living (college, home, etc.).

Most people with a NMD meet criteria for SSI and SSDI based on their diagnosis. Hopefully, patients have been enrolled as children and have been receiving these benefits since close to the time of their diagnosis. If not, families should be directed to resources to help them register. Qualification for SSI varies by state, but in general, one can be eligible with a diagnosis that significantly limits function and/or if a person meets certain income requirements. As patients approach their 18th birthday, they will need to be prepared to undergo a benefit review to see if they remain eligible for SSI. The patient's childhood condition may fall under Medical Listing/Blue Book and automatically denote qualification, or the review may need to demonstrate severity to meet listing to qualify. For this review, SSI officials usually need medical records for the prior year, and medical providers can also offer a letter of support in the application [10]. In most states, if an individual qualifies for SSI, they also qualify for Medicaid insurance coverage. Many of these patients may also qualify for SSDI benefits, but these are limited to citizens who have a work history. Again, patients need to meet certain medical requirements [9]. SSDI coverage is particularly helpful for patients who are able to work part of their adult lives but lose the ability to maintain gainful employment due to progression of disease. These patients should be directed to start the SSDI process as soon as unable to work, as a waiting period exists for benefits to start. After 24 months of receiving benefits and the waiting period (total of 29 months), patients are also eligible to start receiving Medicare benefits. A few conditions automatically qualify for Medicare, with ALS being most relevant to this population [42]. There are certain supports as well as restrictions for patients receiving SSI and SSDI benefits with regard to the level of gainful employment in which they can engage while still receiving benefits, and patients to whom this applies should be familiar with these earning caps. Below are some potentially helpful links:

- www.ssa.gov
- https://www.ssa.gov/benefits/disability/
- https://www.ssa.gov/disability/professionals/bluebook/general-info.htm
- ACA US Department of Health and Human Services, https://www.health-care.gov/, https://www.hhs.gov/healthcare/about-the-aca/index.html
- https://www.hhs.gov/answers/medicare-and-medicaid/who-is-elibible-for-medicare/index.html

Many of the conditions causing neuromuscular disability also entail neuropsychiatric conditions, some involving changes to cognitive function [4], such as frontotemporal dementia/executive function changes in amyotrophic lateral sclerosis (ALS) and potential cognitive involvement in cerebral palsy (CP) [19]. Others have strong associations, such as autism spectrum disorder (ASD) and attention-deficit/ hyperactivity disorder (ADHD), in DMD [29]. Many patients will also experience secondary effects of their condition. In the setting of medical complexity and dependence on multiple devices and treatments, frequent hospitalizations, and experiencing childhood as a chronically ill person, many adolescents and young adults have delayed psychosocial development and maturity [14, 26]. An important role of transition planning is to educate patients and families about steps toward independence and enforce practices that enable patients to take over their own care (talk directly to patients, interview independently, graded ownership of care and medical information). For some, dedicated efforts to facilitate independence are able to help them attain a desired level of independence. For others, "full independence" in the traditional sense is not a realistic goal, and an optimistic but realistic approach to their goals is needed [4]. It is very important to discuss with patients and parents what their goal adulthood looks like. Some patients will desire as "normal" of a life as possible, while others will be very content with graded independence. The traditional view of achieving independent adulthood may or may not apply, and providers need to keep an open mind in discussing what matters most to patients, then focusing on these goals as better markers of optimized outcomes.

Many patients/families will also need to address guardianship, which primarily refers to appointing a person(s) to make medical decisions for someone (sometimes employed along with conservatorship, which primarily refers to a legally appointed person responsible for the financial decisions of an impaired individual). The need for guardianship should be assessed early on in adolescence, as the process requires time, and can be much more challenging after the patient has reached adulthood. Guardianship is a parallel concept to competency, both being legal designations of whether or not an individual can make their own decisions. Capacity, on the other hand, can be fluid and case-by-case with different decisions/situations. This can be assessed by clinical providers and can change day to day. To have capacity, the patient needs to be able to understand the risk/benefit/alternative of treatment options and reason with this information to make and communicate their decision. It is important to establish wishes, roles, and documentation before an emergency arises that limits capacity. Shared decision-making should be used whenever possible if independent decision-making is not feasible (*disability*). Legal support varies by state, but assistance can be found through Supported Decision-Making, ACLU Disability Rights Program, and National Resource Center for Supported Decision-Making, or the Quality Trust for Individuals with Disabilities. If guardianship is warranted, this process is completed through a petition to the court, and the specifics vary by state. Through the National Guardianship Association, one can look for state organizations which can help navigate the process, as well as when and how to start. Whenever possible, patient preferences, input, and autonomy should be respected, and patient autonomy should be preserved as much as possible. Below are resources that may be helpful:

- supporteddecisionmaking.org – National Resource Center for Supported Decision-Making
- dcqualitytrust.org – Quality Trust for Individuals with Disabilities
- www.guardianship.org – National Guardianship Association

While some patients may be able to reach full independence, or nearly so, most will still have some dependence on caregivers. An additional consideration as patients age through adolescence and young adulthood is that their caregivers, often parents, are also aging and facing their own medical and functional changes. Caregiver responsibilities may be taken over by paid caregivers, other family members or friends, or a significant other of the patient. This change can be challenging emotionally, logistically, and financially for both patients and caregivers. Providers can help patients and families navigate these situations again by relying on multidisciplinary support from social workers [30] and counselors/mental health providers and by giving dedicated attention to these topics in transition planning visits. Parents and primary caregivers should be counseled to consider their child's long-term care in estate planning and should arrange for caregivers/support in case of unexpected death or debility.

Social/Emotional/Functional Aspects

As part of normal development, patients progress through stages to become independent from their parents and caregivers. This complex process may be delayed when these patients are dependent for many of their activities of daily living and may be further complicated when the patients have cognitive deficits [4]. In *Living with MD1*, the mother of four patients with myotonic dystrophy 1 details the struggles that her sons and daughter went through during their adolescence and those that persist into adulthood [43]. Patients with this condition (or other NMD) may desire to have normal friendships and romantic relationships despite being dependent for activities of daily living and needing to use positive pressure ventilation at night. Relationships can be particularly challenging when the patient has a disease that will be life-limiting [18, 41]. Some patients have joined condition-specific support groups online that help patients navigate daily life. Support groups can be helpful for caregivers as they navigate the complex medical world. Social workers can be helpful for providing further local and national resources. This aspect of growth and development in AYA with NMD highlights the importance of supportive medical and social environments, as well as an area of life that contributes greatly to quality of life and warrants adequate mental health and medical support.

It can be challenging for providers to help patients become more independent both socially and medically. Got Transition recommends that when the patient reaches age 12, joint discussions should begin with patients and caregivers to plan these transitions. Taking responsibility for their own medical care is an important step for some patients, while others may not have the cognitive or physical capability to take complete responsibility for their medical care.

The subject of our case study has significant mobility issues and requires caregiver assistance with some activities of daily living such as wheelchair transfers. She noted that her parents taught her to be a vocal advocate for her care even though she was not able to do everything herself. She had hired caregivers and trained them with proper protocols. She reports that doing this at a young age gave her confidence and control over her condition. Importantly, she was able to standardize her care between caregivers. One of her challenges with transitioning to college was transportation. She uses a motorized wheelchair and the bus transportation system, but some portions of roads and sidewalks were difficult to navigate. She also had difficulty with new buildings that could not accommodate her wheelchair. This required considerable advanced planning to adapt to the university environment. Furthermore, upgrading and adjusting her wheelchair as needed has been a challenge with insurance coverage.

Her transition also entailed the challenge of hiring new qualified caregivers. She was able to hire students from a local nursing school, and they in return gained experience and were compensated for their services. She is a very bright student and did well academically in high school. She was interested in journalism study for college. Prior to selecting her university, she inquired about accommodations for both physical and academic options. She needed more time for transportation around campus because some buses did not have wheelchair capability. Location of classes was also important because she would need to find elevator access and adequate room for her wheelchair. She also felt mobility and access was key for being able to socialize with other students and to feel like she was a part of the community. She wanted to be as independent as possible and succeed like other students. Sometimes these challenges would be difficult and our patient would struggle emotionally. She contacted the clinic social worker for support and was able to receive counseling, although the first recommendation she received was for a counselor in a building that was not wheelchair accessible.

Successful transition for a number of patients requires using resources such as counseling, social work, and in some cases palliative care. Pediatric palliative care has had different models, depending on location and institution. Palliative care on the adult side is often used when patients are within 6 months of death or making difficult care decisions. It has been observed that pediatric palliative care patients are followed more long-term and for more symptom management. Early and consistent involvement of palliative care (via primary providers or a consulting specialty team) can help to address psychosocial distress as well as physical symptoms of disease and treatment. Early involvement also is known to enhance quality of life and minimize aggressive end of life interventions when not consistent with patient goals [35]. Additionally, these patients benefit from extra support in developing coping skills in the face of progressive illness [41]. Palliative care providers receive extra training to help manage symptoms and support quality of life while adequately supporting the patient's developing psychosocial abilities and needs.

In the multidisciplinary clinics at the University of Michigan and at the University of Utah, we have used a combination of social workers, psychiatrists, therapists, and palliative care to cover the spectrum of needs. On average about 16 patients per year transitioned from pediatric providers to the adult clinic (personal communication from the author). Advanced planning is needed for major life decisions and for facing the reality of aging caregivers. Institutional support is key in providing resources. Full-time equivalents can be shared between different clinics to help support the cost of these providers and support staff. The resources skilled support staff (such as dieticians, care managers, PT/OT, etc.) provide for these patients and providers are invaluable.

Medical Transition

Ideally, the care environment for adults with neuromuscular disease would mirror that of pediatric multidisciplinary clinics. Though data in this area is sparse, patients with NMD do tend to have better outcomes and higher levels of societal function if involved in a multidisciplinary clinical environment [5, 38, 41]. If that is not possible, close communication between the pediatric and adult providers including social work and palliative care is key. Changes in equipment may also happen with pediatric to adult transition, such as tracheostomy placement, for patients that use invasive ventilation. An otolaryngology provider could follow them long-term or they may need a new provider. New insurance coverage and new DME companies will often be part of the transition as well. One example we have noted is that vest therapy, as a mucus clearance device, is favored more frequently for pediatric patients than adult patients.

As these patients transition, there also needs to be planning discussions about general health and function, including reproductive health. A genetic counselor could be helpful for this as well. Mental health support is extremely important and also an inadequately addressed area of wellbeing for these patients [20, 41]. Aside from multiple issues specific to the NMD involved [6], AYA patients still need the normal screening and counseling appropriate for their age group, which can usually be managed by an involved primary care provider within the multidisciplinary medical home or in the community [34, 45].

Transition Stages/Process

Got Transition is a national program focused on healthcare transition with many helpful resources that are easily accessible online from the homepage of gottransition.org. It is a cooperative agreement between the National Alliance to Advance Adolescent Health and the Maternal and Child Health Bureau. The content of Got Transition is aimed to serve healthcare providers, patients, and families. Within the website are several documents to support providers in making a transition policy, tracking individual progress during the process as well as assessing readiness and planning for transition, carrying out the actual transition to adult providers, welcome/orientation visits, and tracking outcomes. There are distinct sets of resources for pediatric providers, accepting adult providers, and those who may be taking care of the patient across the life span (i.e., family medicine or internal medicine-pediatrics-trained physicians). Got Transition also has information about provider education and many patient topics such as guardianship, insurance, education/employment, and resources for patients. This is an excellent resource for providers, patients, and families and contains a well-curated body of information for reference and program development with much of the content also available in Spanish [17].

Starting around age 12, patients should enter into the transition process. Initial discussions can involve introduction of a transition policy, which generally includes when and how this process happens in clinic, as well as expectations and goals for providers, parents, and patients. During the transition process, patients then perform repeated self-assessments to assess readiness and progress. Over time, patients should proceed stepwise through a checklist adapted to the clinic and to the patient's specific needs and disease process. It is expected that this process will take several years, and variability between patients is also to be expected. Written (or electronic) self-assessments during clinic visits can allow patients and providers to monitor objective changes over time as patients progress in their readiness. It is time to formulate a plan for the actual transition to adult care once a patient (1) has completed the checklist or is nearing completion, (2) has a good understanding of their medical situation and needs, and (3) is progressing in self-care and self-advocacy skills (monitored by self-assessments). The patient then needs to gather a medical summary, including plans of care centered on patient goals, prepare an emergency plan, identify adult providers, and schedule first visits with those providers. Such a plan will require substantial individualized adaptation for patients with intellectual disability or severe functional impairments. Providers and parents should be discussing more global issues such as guardianship/conservatorship, adult insurance coverage, and disability benefits early in the process, whether or not the patient is ready to participate and fully understand these topics. These conversations should not be put off until the year or two prior to transition. Assessment of and action in these areas should be addressed early and often in the transition process [17].

Logistically, the clinic office managing a transition will need digital or paper files containing assessments, checklists, legal and insurance documentation, and medical summaries. It may be beneficial to provide a set of this information for patients as well to allow them to track their own progress and gain skills in self-management. Clinics may benefit from a database of all patients involved in the transition process to allow for rapid, efficient check-ins on clinic-wide progress and needs. Some clinics may also benefit from dedicated transition clinic days where multidisciplinary transition team efforts can be focused in a dedicated clinic environment. It is important for members of the transition care team to have clearly designated roles for specific areas of transition, such as selecting adult providers including subspecialists and making appointments, addressing education and vocational goals, managing insurance, etc., to reduce redundancy in clinical time and efforts. Documentation may be aided by formatting templates in the electronic medical record that can be edited and seen by all members of the team or paper or electronic tracking sheets shared by providers. At each routine visit during the transition period, progress should be evaluated and interventions tailored as needed to keep patients on track to transition between ages 18 and 22. It should be noted that not all patients fit this structure; depending on severity of illness and prognosis, some patients may be better served by remaining with their pediatric providers, particularly if life expectancy would not yield the patient experience to be best served by establishing new providers at the end of life.

Throughout the process, providers should make intentional efforts to include the patient directly in interviews and decision-making. This includes eye contact while speaking, directing questions to the patient, and interviewing independently for at least part of every visit. The goal of these adaptations to the classic parent-centered style of interviewing, prevalent in pediatrics, is to gradually empower the patient to take more ownership of their health and needs and to learn to speak for themselves. These skills will be invaluable in the adult care setting, as well as in efforts to maximally function in education, work, and social settings. Parents may need encouragement to allow their children to take over in this manner, and the provider is in an excellent place to set expectations and gently encourage graduated patient autonomy.

Several models of these assessments, checklists, medical summaries, and emergency plans are available from various transition support programs. One well-tailored to this population can be found in the Transition Toolkit for DMD supplementary materials: Readiness Assessment, Checklist, Medical Summary [39]. This resource has documents specifically adapted for patients with DMD, which will address the needs of many patients in the NMD world and provides a thorough outline for adaptations to patients with other neuromuscular disorders. Additionally, free sample documents are available to download from the Got Transition website. These are available in groupings specific to providers facilitating pediatric to adult care transfer, the receiving adult providers, and those who will have continuity but need to adjust care as patients grow (family medicine and internal medicine-pediatrics). Documents are much more generic to suit the needs of patients with a whole host of conditions but can be adapted to specific patient needs. The Got Transition materials also have a wealth of information about developing a general transition clinic policy and process. Clinics that care for patients with chronic neuromuscular respiratory failure would be advised to create their own templates using the resources above, including the child neurology transition checklist example [17, 37].

In preparing patients to transfer to adult care and potentially into more independent environments in other areas of life, providers have a unique opportunity to outfit patients with an effective emergency plan. This can be helpful at any age or stage of illness but is particularly useful if the patient is away from primary caregivers and medical institutions. Patients should have easy, constant access to pertinent medical information at all times in case of emergency. This should include, at minimum, primary medical conditions, allergies, medications, and any emergency plans specific to their condition that may be unfamiliar to community providers. This information can be in a number of formats – a pocket card with relevant medical details, a phone application (e.g., Medical ID is already standard on iPhone or Android), or a digital copy of a medical summary on phone or in email. The Got Transition website and Toolkit for DMD supplementary documents provide excellent guidance for what to include. There is also an emergency pocket card available from the Got Transition resources page. Providers should also address the hospital of choice at the patient's primary location (may change with school, moving) [17].

Once the patient has transitioned into the adult clinic setting, referring and accepting providers have an excellent opportunity to collect feedback and outcomes data to guide improvements to the transition process. Phone interviews, written or online evaluations, and dedicated conversations during clinic visits can yield invaluable insight into the patient and family experience of the transition process and inform providers on areas for improvement and success. Objective outcomes data can also provide much needed evidence to the field of transition medicine, in general, and to this population in neuromuscular disorders, specifically. Several different areas of medicine have small studies of parent-patient-provider feedback in the transition process, which may be helpful in formulating new studies specific to NMD [28, 32].

Potentially Helpful Resources
- People-Process-Performance from MDA, https://strongly.mda.org/the-three-ps-of-transitioning-from-pediatric-to-adult-clinical-care/
- https://gottransition.org/providers/index.cfm
- www.childneurologyfoundation.org/transitions

There are many different models in the world of transition medicine, which are ever-changing and adapting to the needs of patients and institutions. Depending on the strengths and needs of a population or institution, providers could consider the following structures as outlines for their own programs:

- Inpatient transition team or consult service. This structure may include an inpatient care team dedicated to patients in the transition age group and attend to their needs with transition planning in mind. The consult service model could allow providers familiar with the process to meet patients during an inpatient stay and help them organize a plan to meet their needs in transitioning providers and potentially institutions.
- Dedicated transition clinic, specifically to address transition readiness and planning and follow patients in the pre- and post-transition phases of their care to provide some continuity in the process. This could be disease specific or available to any AYA with medical complexity.
- Creating a day or half day specifically set aside for patients in the ages of transition preparation or action, which could be specific in a disease process (i.e., spina bifida clinic or Duchenne clinic) or a general location with support staff to allow various specialties and conditions to utilize the environment (i.e., Tuesday PM genetics, Wednesday AM NMD, Friday PM DM1).
- A planned follow-up visit or contact (email, phone, etc.) after the first appointment(s) with adult providers to assess for additional needs or areas for improvement in the process (i.e., Do you feel comfortable with your new provider? How could we make the process better?)
- Establish a continuity provider who will remain with the patient through the transition to adult subspecialists and is comfortable and able to assist in this process (i.e., primary care provider in family medicine or internal medicine-pediatrics, social worker, cross-trained respiratory therapist).
- Identify a provider in your group who will handle all of the outgoing or incoming transition patients in your practice. This could consolidate resources and experience in a narrower set of clinic staff.

Summary with Areas for Progress

Over the past couple of decades, substantial advancements in disease-specific therapies and chronic condition management have drastically changed the patient experience with many NMDs. This has created incredible opportunities for patients and families, as well as new frontiers and challenges for the medical teams caring for these patients. There is ample opportunity for research in many different areas, particularly with regard to quality improvement in provider education and the transition process [3, 41]. We have minimal data to guide interventions; any contributions of research, care models, treatment strategies, or institutional policy can be helpful in cultivating best practices in the ever-changing care of patients with NMDs. Continuing medical education has a vital role to play on both pediatric and adult sides, but special focus on augmenting education and training in these previously pediatric-specific disease processes for adult-trained providers is warranted [22, 40]. As a medical system, we have a prime opportunity to work to improve the outcomes and experiences of AYA with chronic health needs [16].

Bibliography

1. A Guide to Disability Rights Laws. 24 Feb 2020. Disponível em: https://www.ada.gov/cguide. htm#anchor62335. Acesso em: 7 Apr.
2. Abbott D, Carpenter J, Bushby K. Transition to adulthood for young men with Duchenne muscular dystrophy: research from the UK. Neuromuscul Disord. 2012;22(5):445–6.
3. Agarwal A, Willis D, Tang X, Bauer M, et al. Transition of respiratory technology dependent patients from pediatric to adult pulmonology care. Pediatr Pulmonol. 2015;50(12):1294–300.
4. Baldanzi S, Ricci G, Simoncini C, Cosci ODCM, et al. Hard ways towards adulthood: the transition phase in young people with myotonic dystrophy. Acta Myol. 2016;35(3):145–9.
5. Bent N, Tennant A, Swift T, Posnett J, et al. Team approach versus ad hoc health services for young people with physical disabilities: a retrospective cohort study. Lancet. 2002;360(9342):1280–6.
6. Bushby K, Finkel R, Birnkrant DJ, Case LE, et al. Diagnosis and management of Duchenne muscular dystrophy, part 1: diagnosis, and pharmacological and psychosocial management. Lancet Neurol. 2010a;9(1):77–93.
7. Bushby K, Finkel R, Birnkrant DJ, Case LE, et al. Diagnosis and management of Duchenne muscular dystrophy, part 2: implementation of multidisciplinary care. Lancet Neurol. Feb 2010b;9(2):177–89.
8. Chatwin M, Tan HL, Bush A, Rosenthal M, et al. Long term non-invasive ventilation in children: impact on survival and transition to adult care. PLoS One. 2015;10(5):e0125839.
9. Disability Benefits. Disponível em: https://www.ssa.gov/benefits/disability/. Acesso em: 7 Apr.
10. Disability Evaluation Under Social Security. Medical/Professional relations. Disponível em: https://www.ssa.gov/disability/professionals/bluebook/general-info.htm. Acesso em: 7 Apr.
11. Disability, U. N. D. O. E. A. S. A. Convention on the Rights of Persons with Disabilities: Article 12 – Equal recognition before the law. Disponível em: https://www.un.org/development/desa/disabilities/convention-on-the-rights-of-persons-with-disabilities/article-12-equal-recognition-before-the-law.html.
12. Duchenne and Becker muscular dystrophy. Your guide to understanding genetic conditions, Genetics Home Reference, NIH, 2020. Acesso em: 7 Apr.
13. Dystrophinopathies. Neuromuscular, Neuromuscular Disease Center, 5/16/19 2019. Disponível em: https://neuromuscular.wustl.edu/musdist/dmd.html. Acesso em: 7 Apr.
14. Evan EE, Zeltzer LK. Psychosocial dimensions of cancer in adolescents and young adults. Cancer. 2006;107(7 Suppl):1663–71.
15. Gloss D, Moxley RT, Ashwal S, Oskoui M. Practice guideline update summary: corticosteroid treatment of Duchenne muscular dystrophy: report of the guideline development Subcommittee of the American Academy of Neurology. In: Neurology, vol. 86; 2016. p. 465–72.
16. Goodman DM, Hall M, Levin A, Watson RS, et al. Adults with chronic health conditions originating in childhood: inpatient experience in children's hospitals. Pediatrics. 2011;128(1):5–13.
17. Got Transition. Disponível em: https://www.gottransition.org/. Acesso em: 7 Apr.

18. Hamdani Y, Mistry B, Gibson BE. Transitioning to adulthood with a progressive condition: best practice assumptions and individual experiences of young men with Duchenne muscular dystrophy. Disabil Rehabil. 2015;37(13):1144–51.
19. Hendriksen JG, Vles JS. Neuropsychiatric disorders in males with Duchenne muscular dystrophy: frequency rate of attention-deficit hyperactivity disorder (ADHD), autism spectrum disorder, and obsessive – compulsive disorder. J Child Neurol. 2008;23(5):477–81.
20. Lindsay S, Mcadam L, Mahendiran T. Enablers and barriers of men with Duchenne muscular dystrophy transitioning from an adult clinic within a pediatric hospital. Disabil Health J. 2017;10(1):73–9.
21. Michelson D, Ciafaloni E, Ashwal S, Lewis E, et al. Evidence in focus: Nusinersen use in spinal muscular atrophy: Report of the Guideline Development, Dissemination, and Implementation Subcommittee of the American Academy of Neurology. Neurology. 2018;91(20):923–33.
22. Mixter S, Stewart RW. Adult head and neck health care needs for individuals with complex chronic conditions of childhood. Med Clin North Am. 2018;102(6):1055–61.
23. Ng SY, Dinesh SK, Tay SK, Lee EH. Decreased access to health care and social isolation among young adults with cerebral palsy after leaving school. J Orthop Surg (Hong Kong). 2003;11(1):80–9.
24. Online Mendelian Inheritance in Man (OMIM). 2020.
25. Passamano L, Taglia A, Palladino A, Viggiano E, et al. Improvement of survival in Duchenne Muscular Dystrophy: retrospective analysis of 835 patients. Acta Myol. 2012;31:121–5.
26. Pinquart M, Teubert D. Academic, physical, and social functioning of children and adolescents with chronic physical illness: a meta-analysis. J Pediatr Psychol. 2012;37(4):376–89.
27. Preutthipan A. Home mechanical ventilation in children. Indian J Pediatr. Sep 2015;82(9):852–9.
28. Rauen K, Sawin KJ, Bartelt T, Waring WP, et al. Transitioning adolescents and young adults with a chronic health condition to adult healthcare - an exemplar program. Rehabil Nurs. 2013;38(2):63–72.
29. Ricotti V, Mandy WP, Scoto M, Pane M, et al. Neurodevelopmental, emotional, and behavioural problems in Duchenne muscular dystrophy in relation to underlying dystrophin gene mutations. Dev Med Child Neurol. 2016;58(1):77–84.
30. Rizzolo MC, Hemp R, Braddock D, Schindler A. Family support services for persons with intellectual and developmental disabilities: recent national trends. Intellect Dev Disabil. 2009;47(2):152–5.
31. Schrans DG, Abbott D, Peay HL, Pangalila RF, et al. Transition in Duchenne muscular dystrophy: an expert meeting report and description of transition needs in an emergent patient population: (Parent Project Muscular Dystrophy Transition Expert Meeting 17–18 June 2011, Amsterdam, The Netherlands). Neuromuscul Disord. 2013;23(3):283–6.
32. Sonneveld HM, Strating MM, Van Staa AL, Nieboer AP. Gaps in transitional care: what are the perceptions of adolescents, parents and providers? Child Care Health Dev. 2013;39(1):69–80.
33. Statute and Regulations. Disponível em: https://sites.ed.gov/idea/statuteregulations/#regulations. Acesso em: 7 Apr.
34. Suris JC, Michaud PA, Akre C, Sawyer SM. Health risk behaviors in adolescents with chronic conditions. Pediatrics. 2008;122(5):e1113–8.
35. Temel JS, Greer JA, Muzikansky A, Gallagher ER, et al. Early palliative care for patients with metastatic non-small-cell lung cancer. N Engl J Med. 2010;363(8):733–42.
36. The Rehabilitation Act of 1973. 10 Dec 2015. Disponível em: https://www2.ed.gov/policy/speced/reg/narrative.html. Acesso em: 7 Apr.
37. Transitions Checklist: Young Adults with Neurologic Disorders. ACT HVC pediatric to adult care transition project. Disponível em: https://www.childneurologyfoundation.org/wp-content/uploads/2017/08/B_TransitionChecklist.pdf. Acesso em: 7 Apr.
38. Traynor BJ, Alexander M, Corr B, Frost E, et al. Effect of a multidisciplinary amyotrophic lateral sclerosis (ALS) clinic on ALS survival: a population based study, 1996-2000. J Neurol Neurosurg Psychiatry. 2003;74(9):1258–61.

39. Trout CJ, Case LE, Clemens PR, Mcarthur A, et al. A transition toolkit for Duchenne muscular dystrophy. Pediatrics. 2018;142(Suppl 2):S110–s117.
40. Van Lierde A, Menni F, Bedeschi MF, Natacci F, et al. Healthcare transition in patients with rare genetic disorders with and without developmental disability: neurofibromatosis 1 and Williams-Beuren syndrome. Am J Med Genet A. 2013;161a(7):1666–74.
41. Wan HWY, Carey KA, D'silva A, Kasparian NA, et al. "Getting ready for the adult world": how adults with spinal muscular atrophy perceive and experience healthcare, transition and well-being. Orphanet J Rare Dis. 2019;14(1):74.
42. Who is eligible for Medicare? Disponível em: https://www.hhs.gov/answers/medicare-and-medicaid/who-is-elibible-for-medicare/index.html. Acesso em: 7 Apr.
43. Woodbury AS. Living with DM1: my family's story. 2017.
44. Young Adult Coverage. About the ACA. Disponível em: https://www.hhs.gov/healthcare/about-the-aca/young-adult-coverage/index.html. Acesso em: 7 Apr.
45. Zbikowski SM, Klesges RC, Robinson LA, Alfano CM. Risk factors for smoking among adolescents with asthma. J Adolesc Health. 2002;30(4):279–87.

Chapter 9
Establishing a Medical Home for Asthma and Other Obstructive Lung Diseases

Nadia L. Krupp and Sarah E. Bauer

Asthma

Preparing the adolescent asthma patient for transition to adult care should include the following:

1. Assessment of the risk of adult asthma
2. Optimization of medical therapy
3. Optimization of lung function by late adolescence
4. Education regarding disease
5. Identification of appropriate adult provider (primary care, allergist, pulmonologist).
6. Accurate description/phenotyping to adult provider

Asthma, like other chronic lung conditions, is multifactorial in terms of inception, severity, and prognosis. The pathogenesis of asthma is complex and involves combinations of genetic, environmental, infectious, and inflammatory factors. Furthermore, over the course of an asthmatic patient's childhood, adolescence, and adulthood, environmental and infectious exposures are in a continuous state of flux. When considering the transition of a patient with asthma from pediatric to adult care, considerations include not only prognosis and pharmacologic needs but also environmental exposure considerations both in the home and in the anticipated workplace.

N. L. Krupp (✉) · S. E. Bauer
Riley Hospital for Children, Division of Pediatric Pulmonology, Allergy and Sleep Medicine, Indianapolis, IN, USA
e-mail: nkrupp@iu.edu

© Springer Nature Switzerland AG 2021
C. D. Brown, E. Crowley (eds.), *Transitioning Care from Pediatric to Adult Pulmonology*, Respiratory Medicine,
https://doi.org/10.1007/978-3-030-68688-8_9

The onset of asthma symptoms can occur at any age, from very early childhood, through adolescence and adulthood. Children with wheezing very early in life can exhibit transient symptoms, rather than lifelong asthma. External factors such as the timing, type, and number of respiratory infections and the constitution and diversity of the airway microbiome can also modulate the natural history, affecting severity as well as persistence of asthma symptoms over the course of years. Parental asthma history, presence of atopic comorbidities, and wheezing outside of viral infections all help predict which trajectory a young child with wheezing is most likely to follow [1].

For children who exhibit asthma symptoms beyond the first few years of life into adolescence, their risk of lifelong asthma is much higher. This is particularly pronounced for children with severe asthma, as the risk of asthma that persists into adulthood is tenfold higher for children and adolescents with severe disease compared to their milder counterparts [2]. Of course, with recent advances in biologic and pharmacologic therapies, the natural history of severe asthma is likely to be ever-changing. Biologic agents and steroid-sparing treatments have the potential to significantly improve symptom control while minimizing medication-related side effects and improving quality of life.

Current Practices in Adolescent to Adult Asthma Transition

There is a paucity of existing research regarding the transition of the patient with asthma from pediatric to adult care and a lack of established best practices for effectively guiding patients with asthma through this process. However, there are some common patterns of care that have emerged over time. Rather than being evidence based, these patterns have evolved due to logistic factors such as insurance coverage, geography, provider availability, and provider experience with asthma medications. As such, further research is needed in order to establish best practices for both the mild to moderate asthma patient and asthma patients with severe disease as they transition to adult care.

At present, adult patients with mild to moderate asthma often have their asthma managed by their primary care provider. However, patients who require biologic therapy or multiple controller medications such as inhaled corticosteroid (ICS), long-acting beta agonist (LABA), and long-acting muscarinic antagonist (LAMA) are more likely to be under the care of an adult asthma specialist, such as an allergist or adult pulmonologist. Considerations in identifying the best adult asthma specialist include geographic, transportation, insurance, and regional considerations as well as the type of therapy involved such as biologic agents or immunotherapy.

Asthma and Lung Function

One advantage of referring adult patients with moderate to severe asthma to an asthma specialist is the availability of lung function testing. An adolescent with severe asthma is much more likely to have a diminished peak in their normal lung growth. Furthermore, a child with severe asthma will have an accelerated decline in lung function throughout adulthood compared to a mild asthmatic or non-asthmatic counterpart. The combination of these two processes means that adolescents with severe asthma who demonstrate persistent obstruction on spirometry have a higher risk of decreased lung function in early adulthood compared to those with milder disease. Similarly, patients in early adulthood with asthma who have persistently abnormal lung function are much more likely to have permanent obstruction throughout adulthood and increased risk of functional impairment [2]. However, even adolescent asthma patients with persistent obstruction on lung function testing have a chance of regaining normal or near-normal lung function by early adulthood. As a result, the teenage years are a critical period for maximizing lung function.

In addition to tracking lung function related to asthma, lung function testing and specialist involvement can provide an opportunity to evaluate for other forms of lung disease that can masquerade as asthma in children and adolescents. Certain rare diseases, such as alpha 1 antitrypsin deficiency, can manifest as asthma-like symptoms in childhood but evolve in early adulthood when the first signs of emphysema can occur. Routine, reliable lung function testing and specialist input can allow for a timely diagnosis in this population.

Medication Considerations for Transition to Adult Care

Soliciting the patient's goals of care is important, ideally as soon as the patient is developmentally able to verbalize such goals, and well before the anticipated transition to adult care. School-aged children can typically describe their goals regarding both lifestyle and health and should be engaged in discussions about their disease and medications as early as possible. In earlier childhood years, conversations with the child will be centered on ensuring the child knows that asthma is a chronic disease and why they may be given medication every day even when they feel well. The school-aged child can often also verbalize their own priorities, which may differ from those of the parent and provider. For example, a parent's goals may be to decrease ED visits and calls from school; the provider's goals may be to optimize lung function and decrease hospitalizations; and the child's goals may be to participate in organized sports and get through an entire game without getting short of breath. All of these goals may align well and be accomplished with the same changes in medications; however, getting engagement from the parent and child on the treatment strategy is best accomplished if their goals are honored, validated, and included in the discussion. Essentially, the child may be more motivated to take their twice-daily controller medication if they view it as their "be able to play a whole game" medicine. Parent and child goals are likely to change over time, so frequently revisiting previously stated goals, and establishing current goals of care is important.

Adherence challenges are augmented in adolescence by a developmentally normal sense of invincibility and immunity from the life-threatening complications of asthma

As the asthma patient transitions through adolescence, conversations should become more in depth and shift focus to the adolescent's ability to care for themselves. Goals, priorities, and attitudes toward chronic disease change frequently during this stage of life, and engaging the patient is at the same time more difficult and more important than ever. The provider can utilize strategies such as shared decision-making and motivational interviewing to engage the patient, solicit their views on asthma management, and address adherence. These approaches help the patient feel more invested in their treatment plan, more comfortable with the medications, and more confident in their ability to execute the prescribed plan.

Adherence is a challenge throughout childhood and adolescence for patients with asthma. However, this is augmented in adolescence when normal cognitive developmental stages bring a sense of invincibility and immunity from the life-threatening complications of asthma. Since asthma for many patients is characterized by long asymptomatic periods, punctuated by unpredictable episodic flares, adherence to a daily regimen is difficult for many teenagers with asthma to prioritize. Furthermore, as the adolescent with asthma approaches adulthood, demands on time and energy become more complex. From a practical standpoint, simplifying the medication regimen through once-daily dosing regimens or combined medication inhalers can be beneficial for the adolescent transitioning to adulthood. If the patient's symptoms are mild, with near-normal lung function, then intermittent dosing with inhaled corticosteroid/bronchodilator combination could be an option to minimize the severity of exacerbations while decreasing the day-to-day burden of care [3].

For the patient with mild to moderate asthma, medication-related issues around the time of transition to adult care are typically focused on controller therapy and device usage. Some asthma medications, particularly ICS and ICS/LABA, are available in multiple forms. However, which inhaled formulations are appropriate for a given patient will depend not only on medication class and dosage but also device technique. As such, the transition from childhood to adolescence to adulthood may bring multiple changes in medication and asthma device, particularly if insurance changes concurrently. Care should be taken at each opportunity to review adherence to the regimen, barriers to adherence, intended dosing frequency, and device technique, preferably using the services of an asthma educator. This is particularly important if medication dosing frequency or inhaler technique changes, in order to ensure that medication delivery is optimized.

Outside of medication changes, though, it is well established that for pediatric and adolescent patients of all ages, inhaler technique degrades over time. This is true for even the most well-intentioned and experienced patients, with only a minority of patients demonstrating accurate inhaler technique [4]. Therefore, even in the absence of a medication change, assessment of adherence and technique is recommended at each opportunity.

Environmental Considerations

Children with asthma often have environmental exposures that are out of their control. Exposure to secondhand and thirdhand smoke, pets, cockroaches, mice, dust mites, mold, poor ventilation, and airborne particulate matter often exacerbates pediatric asthma and increases morbidity. The transition to adulthood can provide an opportunity to educate the patient about future life choices that could help decrease their adult symptoms. For example, identification of sensitization to animals may help guide the patient's decision about whether to own a pet or which pets to avoid. Similarly, an asthma patient with sensitization to cats or dogs may be more educated to inquire about previous inhabitants of a home or apartment and choose hard flooring surfaces rather than carpet.

When it comes to occupation, counseling the adolescent about future employment choices can also be informed by their lung disease. If a patient has sensitivity to cold air, for example, then employment in which they are outside in cold winter weather may not be the best choice. Similarly, patients may need to steer away from occupations that involve dust, fumes, aerosols, or facilities that allow indoor smoking.

Communication to Adult Provider

Factors that should be communicated to the adult provider include, but are not limited to, the patient's severity of asthma, medication therapies, and asthma phenotype. This is particularly true for the severe asthmatic for whom the following information would be useful for the accepting adult provider, if known:

Severe adolescent asthma – Factors to communicate to adult provider
- Asthma phenotype
  - Allergic status and known triggers
  - Serum IgE, blood eosinophil count

- Type of airway inflammation (eosinophilic, neutrophilic, paucigran-ulocytic)
- Smoking/substance use history
- Physical and mental health comorbidities

• Current medication regimen

- Recent adherence (and previous challenges)
- Prior therapies and reasons stopped (lack of efficacy, side effects)

• Lung function

- Lowest and highest spirometry values
- Highest post-bronchodilator spirometry values in the last 12–24 months prior to transition
- Patient perception of airway obstruction

    Poor perception increases risk of respiratory failure and asthma related death

• Exacerbation risk

- Seasonality of asthma symptoms
- Systemic steroid exposure in the last 12 months
- Exacerbation type (e.g., rapid decompensation vs symptomatic with slight change in lung function, etc.)
- History of respiratory failure/intubation (lifetime)

Asthma and Chronic Obstructive Pulmonary Disease (COPD)

The presence of severe asthma in adolescence with persistently low baseline lung function increases the future risk of COPD. However, the presence of seemingly fixed obstruction in an adolescent should not be prematurely diagnosed as COPD. Rather, the adolescent lung has the remarkable capacity to normalize lung function with some adolescents demonstrating moderate to severe obstruction consistently, even with a relatively limited bronchodilator response, only to achieve normal or near-normal lung function in early adulthood. This improvement may be due to change in living situation, removal of exposures in the home, improved adherence with maturity, or some combination thereof.

For those severe asthmatics who do have persistent obstruction into adulthood, they may exhibit Asthma-COPD Overlap Syndrome (ACOS). In the presence of severe asthma in a young adult, the inability to achieve normal lung function with aggressive asthma control in between exacerbations may raise the suspicion of future development of COPD or ACOS. However, at this time, a consensus for the definition of ACOS and most appropriate treatment for this complex disease state are still forthcoming [5, 6].

Asthma and Pregnancy

Female patients with severe asthma should be counseled regarding the risk of pregnancy in light of their lung disease. The effects of pregnancy on lung capacity are well known. However, young women with moderate to severe asthma prior to pregnancy will likely have increased dyspnea and potentially an increased tendency for bronchospasm and exacerbations. For patients with severe asthma, a maternal fetal medicine expert should be enlisted to ensure optimization of lung function while minimizing medication exposures to the fetus. This is particularly important for patients who have needed daily oral corticosteroid therapy, oral theophylline, or biologic agents that could cross the placenta and have effects on the fetus.

Bronchopulmonary Dysplasia

Bronchopulmonary dysplasia (BPD) is a chronic respiratory disease that affects individuals born prematurely. Despite continued advances in care, BPD remains one of the most common sequelae of premature birth. Numerous antenatal and postnatal factors can contribute to the complex etiology and pathophysiology of BPD. The diverse combination of causes, such as arrest and impairment of airway and lung development, lung injury, persistent inflammation, abnormal pulmonary vascular development, as well as other genetic and environmental factors, contribute to the heterogeneous group of clinical phenotypes seen in BPD.

As our understanding of the etiology and pathophysiology of BPD has evolved over time, so have the definition and disease severity classifications. To date, there is no one unifying consensus for the definition of BPD. One of the simplest definitions defines BPD as having an oxygen requirement for greater or equal to 28 days from birth to 36 weeks postmenstrual age (PMA). In 2016 the National Institute of Child Health and Human Development (NICHD) proposed a revised definition of BPD which reclassified severity based on a grade system (I, II, III, IIIA) and better accounted for the advances in noninvasive ventilatory technology and death prior to 36 weeks PMA [7]. Per the 2016 NICHD definition, an infant meets the diagnostic criteria for BPD if they were born prior to completing 32 weeks gestational age and have persistent parenchymal lung disease, radiologic confirmation of parenchymal lung disease, and at 36 weeks PMA require supplemental respiratory support for greater or equal than 3 consecutive days to maintain arterial oxygen saturation in the 90–95% range. Depending on the degree of respiratory support and FiO_2 an infant requires at 36 weeks PMA, the infant is classified as grade I, II, or III. If death secondary to persistent parenchymal lung disease and respiratory failure that cannot be attributed to other neonatal morbidities occurs between 14 days postnatal age and 36 weeks PMA, then the infant is classified as grade III(A). However, this definition, nor other diagnostic criteria for BPD, does not always accurately reflect lung function, morbidity, or mortality later in life.

Individuals born extremely premature (EP, less than 28 weeks gestational age) and/or with extremely low birth weight (ELBW, birth weight less than 1000 grams), particularly those with a history of BPD, have lower lung functions and worse airflow obstruction compared to their peers in childhood, adolescence, and into adulthood [8]. They also tend to have more respiratory symptoms and are at higher risk for hospitalization. Normally, forced vital capacity (FVC) and forced expiratory volume in the first second (FEV1) increases throughout childhood, plateaus around 20–25 years of age, and then steadily declines. Studies suggest that individuals born EP/ELBW, particularly those with a history of BPD, do not reach their full airway growth potential. As a result, even if their rate of respiratory decline remains normal, they are at higher risk for development of COPD later in life.

Once discharged from the neonatal intensive care unit (NICU), there are limited guidelines for the outpatient management of BPD. Of the guidelines currently available, most recommendations are based on a low quality of evidence or expert consensus. It is largely agreed upon that a multidisciplinary approach to follow-up should be adapted. Promotion of optimal growth and nutrition is important. Education should be provided with respect to smoking avoidance and cessation, including electronic cigarettes (e-cigarettes), and immunizations, including annual influenza vaccination.

BPD is a chronic lung disease with natural progression that continues through the neonatal period, into childhood, and well into adolescence and adulthood. Adolescents and young adults are at high risk for fractured care and being lost to follow-up. Currently, there is very little to no guidance for, or research on, best practices for long-term follow-up for this patient population. As such, it is imperative to continue to grow and develop multidisciplinary programs as well as support research to better facilitate follow-up, transition, and long-term treatment.

In summary, BPD is a complex multifactorial chronic lung disease. As our understanding of the etiology, pathophysiology, and natural disease course of BPD continues to evolve, so do the diagnostic criteria and management guidelines. What we do know is that children with BPD have decreased lung functions compared to their peers, impaired lung structure, and abnormal vasculature. They also often have other concurrent comorbidities such as, but not limited to, neurodevelopmental impairment, pulmonary hypertension, and poor growth and nutrition. These sequelae of premature birth and BPD contribute to the failure to reach airway growth potential leading to earlier lung function decline and increased respiratory symptoms in adulthood. Thus, for individuals with a history of premature birth and/or BPD, continued multidisciplinary follow-up through childhood and into adulthood, anticipatory guidance, and education is crucial.

Primary Ciliary Dyskinesia and Non-Cystic Fibrosis Bronchiectasis

Primary ciliary dyskinesia (PCD) and non-cystic fibrosis bronchiectasis (NCFB) are predominantly disorders of airway clearance and chronic infection/inflammation. For the adolescents transitioning to adult care with these disorders, a focus on the incorporation of airway clearance into their adult lifestyle is imperative. For example, a high school schedule may allow for vest therapy three times a day, but if, as an adult, the patient will have three or four 10–12-hour shifts per week, then that schedule may not be feasible. Flexibility in daily expectations or incorporation of more portable airway clearance modalities such as handheld devices or autogenic drainage should be considered [9].

Due to the complexity and nuance related to the care of these disorders, care of bronchiectasis in the adult patient should be provided with the input of an adult pulmonologist. Communication to the adult pulmonologist should include the following from the last 2 years: radiographic reports and images of chest imaging, respiratory microbiology, airway clearance regimen, hospitalization history, and spirometry.

Other Obstructive Lung Diseases

Sickle Cell Disease

Sickle cell disease (SCD) refers to a group of inherited disorders characterized by mutations in the gene that encodes the hemoglobin subunit β. This includes sickle cell anemia, sickle beta thalassemia, hemoglobin SC disease, and others. From a pulmonary standpoint, complications of SCD include acute chest syndrome, pulmonary hypertension, asthma and lower airway disease, sleep disordered breathing, hypoxia, thromboembolic disease, and pulmonary fibrosis. Cardiopulmonary complications are a major risk factor for accelerated morbidity and cause of mortality in patients with SCD. Despite this, our understanding of the natural history of SCD-associated pulmonary disease and our knowledge of specific genetic factors and/or comorbidities that increase the risk for cardiopulmonary complications in SCD is significantly limited [10].

The onset of respiratory complications is variable. As such, the involvement of a pulmonologist in the care of a patient with SCD is highly variable across the age range and among different care intuitions. However, it is important to recognize that transition from pediatric to adult care for individuals with SCD is a critical time and is associated with increased utilization of health care as well as increased morbidity and mortality. Pulmonologists should continue to work closely with these individuals, their famil5es, and the rest of their SCD care team to help facilitate a smooth transition.

Others

A number of other obstructive lung diseases are cared for by pediatric pulmonologists which warrant continued care in adult pulmonology. These include but are not limited to bronchiolitis obliterans and anatomic airway anomalies. Transition for such etiologies should be dealt with on a case-to-case basis.

Summary

In summary, asthma and other obstructive lung diseases encountered by pediatric pulmonary physicians such as BPD, PCD, non-cystic fibrosis bronchiectasis, sickle cell disease, and others encompass a wide range of clinical phenotypes and disease severities which persist into adulthood. For these patients, a smooth, well-communicated transition from pediatric to adult pulmonology is imperative to maintain continued care and prevent loss to follow-up.

References

1. Castro-Rodriguez JA, et al. A clinical index to define risk of asthma in young children with recurrent wheezing. Am J Respir Crit Care Med. 2000;162(4 Pt 1):1403–6.
2. Tai A, et al. Outcomes of childhood asthma to the age of 50 years. J Allergy Clin Immunol. 2014;133(6):1572–8.e3.
3. Global Initiative for Asthma. Global strategy for asthma management and prevention; 2019.
4. Sleath B, et al. Provider demonstration and assessment of child device technique during pediatric asthma visits. Pediatrics. 2011;127(4):642–8.
5. Bonten TN, et al. Defining asthma-COPD overlap syndrome: a population-based study. Eur Respir J. 2017;49(5):1602008.
6. Postma DS, Rabe KF. The asthma-COPD overlap syndrome. N Engl J Med. 2015;373(13):1241–9.
7. Higgins RD, et al. Bronchopulmonary dysplasia: executive summary of a workshop. J Pediatr. 2018;197:300–8.
8. Doyle LW, et al. Airway obstruction in young adults born extremely preterm or extremely low birth weight in the postsurfactant era. Thorax. 2019;74(12):1147–53.
9. de Souza Simoni LH, et al. Acute effects of oscillatory PEP and thoracic compression on secretion removal and impedance of the respiratory system in non-cystic fibrosis bronchiectasis. Respir Care. 2019;64(7):818–27.
10. Ruhl AP, et al. Identifying clinical and research priorities in sickle cell lung disease. An official American Thoracic Society workshop report. Ann Am Thorac Soc. 2019;16(9):e17–32.

Chapter 10
Pulmonary Hypertension: Transition Challenges in the Current Therapeutic Era

Jordan D. Awerbach and Wayne J. Franklin

Definition and Classification

Pulmonary hypertension (PH) is a general term describing elevated resting pulmonary arterial pressures (PAP) from any cause. Historically, PH has been defined by a mean PAP (mPAP) $\geq$ 25 mmHg on cardiac catheterization [1]. There has always been recognition that this cutoff, which has been used for nearly 50 years, was chosen somewhat arbitrarily. A systematic review by Kovacs et al. demonstrated that mPAP in normal subjects at rest was 14.0 ± 3.3 mmHg with an upper limit of normal of 20.6 mmHg [2]. Over time it has become increasingly clear that mPAPs of 21–24 mmHg are associated with an increased risk of progression to pulmonary arterial hypertension (PAH) and worsened survival [3–6]. This culminated in the redefinition of PH as a mPAP > 20 mmHg at the 6th World Symposium on Pulmonary Hypertension (WSPH) in 2018 [3].

PH may be further characterized based on whether the cause of elevated pulmonary pressures exists before or after the pulmonary capillary bed. Hemodynamically, pre- versus post-capillary PH is defined by a normal versus elevated pulmonary capillary wedge pressure (PCWP), respectively, which is used as a surrogate for the left atrial pressure. It is important to note that pre- and post-capillary PH may coexist in the same patient. Pulmonary arterial hypertension (PAH) refers to a subset of PH patients with purely pre-capillary disease. PAH is a rare disease marked by vasoconstriction and progressive endothelial dysfunction of the pulmonary vascular bed, leading to pathologic remodeling that results in the obliteration of the pulmonary vasculature and increased pulmonary vascular resistance [7]. This ultimately leads to right heart failure and death. The criteria for diagnosing

J. D. Awerbach (✉) · W. J. Franklin
Phoenix Children's Hospital, Department of Cardiology, Phoenix, AZ, USA
e-mail: jawerbach@phoenixchildrens.com

© Springer Nature Switzerland AG 2021
C. D. Brown, E. Crowley (eds.), *Transitioning Care from Pediatric to Adult Pulmonology*, Respiratory Medicine,
https://doi.org/10.1007/978-3-030-68688-8_10

PAH includes a mPAP > 20 mmHg (previously ≥ 25 mmHg), a PCWP ≤ 15 mmHg, and an elevated pulmonary vascular resistance (PVR) > 3 Wood units (Wu). In children, PVR is typically indexed to body surface area and is elevated >3 Wood units × m2 (iWu) [1, 8]. In 2011, the Pulmonary Vascular Research Institute (PVRI) introduced the term *pulmonary hypertensive vascular disease*, in an effort to better characterize patients with congenital heart disease (CHD) who have undergone single ventricle palliation [9]. The PVRI proposed that pulmonary vascular disease be defined in this group as a PVR > 3 iWu or a transpulmonary gradient >6 mmHg. Elevated mPAP was not included in the definition, as this population may have clinically significant pre-capillary PH in the face of lower pulmonary pressures.

In both children and adults, PH may occur as a primary illness (i.e., idiopathic PAH) or develop secondary to other disease states. The current World Health Organization (WHO) classification system for PH contains five clinical categories representing groupings of disease processes that share common clinical characteristics and PH pathophysiology (Table 10.1). When originally designed, the WHO classification was based on PH-causing diseases seen in the adult population. Numerous modifications to the WHO classification scheme have occurred since its initial creation at the second WSPH (Evian 1998) [10]. A Pediatric Task Force was formed at the fifth WSPH (Nice 2013), at which time modifications were proposed to better incorporate pediatric disorders associated with PH. With an increasing number of pediatric PH patients now surviving into adulthood, these changes recognized the importance of having a common classification system for all patients that would better facilitate a patient's transition into the adult care setting [11]. At the most recent WSPH (Nice 2018), additional pediatric-focused modifications were made to the WHO classification, such as the inclusion of developmental lung disorders (WHO Group 3.5) and separate designations for CHD associated with PAH (Group 1.4.4), CHD with post-capillary PH (Group 2.4), and complex CHD (Group 5.4) [12].

Epidemiology

PH is a heterogeneous disease associated with numerous underlying disorders. There is a significant variability in the distribution of these disorders throughout the world. For example, schistosomiasis affects at least 200 million people and is a leading cause of PH worldwide; however 85% of those affected live in sub-Saharan Africa [13, 14]. As such, characterizing the global incidence and prevalence of all-cause PH is challenging. In a large population-based study of Ontario, Canada, Wijeratne and colleagues reported an annual incidence of PH of 24.1 patients per 100,000 persons and that the prevalence of adult and pediatric PH was 127.3 and 57.9 per 100,000 persons, respectively [15]. There are also important differences in the distribution of PH-causing diseases between pediatric and adult patients (Fig. 10.1). PAH (Group 1) is the most common subgroup of PH seen in children,

Table 10.1 The World
Health Organization
classification system for
pulmonary hypertension
(Nice 2018)

1 *PAH*
1.1 Idiopathic PAH
1.2 Heritable PAH
1.3 Drug- and toxin-induced PAH
1.4 PAH associated with:
1.4.1 Connective tissue disease
1.4.2 HIV infection
1.4.3 Portal hypertension
1.4.4 Congenital heart disease
1.4.5 Schistosomiasis
1.5 PAH long-term responders to calcium channel blockers
1.6 PAH with overt features of venous/capillary (PVOD/PCH) involvement
1.7 Persistent PH of the newborn syndrome
2 *PH due to left heart disease*
2.1 PH due to heart failure with preserved LVEF
2.2 PH due to heart failure with reduced LVEF
2.3 Valvular heart disease
2.4 Congenital/acquired cardiovascular conditions leading to post-capillary PH
3 *PH due to lung diseases and/or hypoxia*
3.1 Obstructive lung disease
3.2 Restrictive lung disease
3.3 Other lung diseases with mixed restrictive/obstructive pattern
3.4 Hypoxia without lung disease
3.5 Developmental lung disorders
4 *PH due to pulmonary artery obstructions*
4.1 Chronic thromboembolic PH
4.2 Other pulmonary artery obstructions
5 *PH with unclear and/or multifactorial mechanisms*
5.1 Hematological disorders
5.2 Systemic and metabolic disorders
5.3 Others
5.4 Complex congenital heart disease

Reproduced with permission of the © ERS 2020: Simonneau
et al. [93]. *Published 24 January 2019*
PAH pulmonary arterial hypertension, *PVOD* pulmonary veno-
occlusive disease, *PCH* pulmonary capillary hemangiomatosis,
LVEF left ventricular ejection fraction

making up 60–90% of registry cohorts [9, 16]. It is also worth noting that PH due to
developmental lung diseases (Group 3) is being seen with increased prevalence, and
this group now represents 10–12% of the pediatric PH population [16–18]. PH in
adults is far more common than PAH and is most often seen in association with

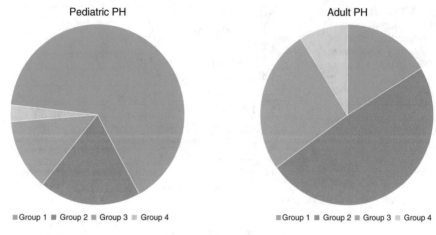

Fig. 10.1 Distribution of PH by the WHO group for pediatric and adult patients seen in a large population-based cohort. (Data taken from [15])

left-sided heart disease (Group 2) and pulmonary disease (Group 1) [7, 16, 19]. Chronic heart failure and chronic obstructive pulmonary disease currently affect 61 million and 250 million adults, respectively, worldwide [13]. All forms of PH have been associated with increased mortality in patients [15, 19].

PAH is a rare disease in both children and adults, with an estimated prevalence of 2–16 cases per million children and 15–60 cases per million adults [1, 7, 20]. A nationwide registry in the Netherlands found the majority of pediatric patients had transient forms of PAH, including persistent pulmonary hypertension of the newborn and flow-related PAH in children with systemic-to-pulmonary shunts (e.g., ventricular septal defect or patent ductus arteriosus) that were reversible after shunt closure [16]. Of the remaining patients with progressive PAH, 72% had CHD and 27% had idiopathic PAH (IPAH). The annual incidence rates for CHD-associated PAH and IPAH were 2.2 and 0.7 cases per million, and the point prevalence was 15.6 and 4.4 cases per million, respectively. The Spanish REHIPED registry reported similar findings; the incidence of IPAH versus CHD-APAH was 0.49 and 1.87 cases per million per year, and the prevalence was 2.9 and 10.1 cases per million, respectively [9]. IPAH makes up a larger proportion of adult PAH patients, representing about half of the cases seen in adult registries [21]. PAH demonstrates a female predominance in both children and adults. In the US REVEAL registry, 80% of adults and 64% of children were female [22, 23].

Prior to the introduction of targeted PAH pharmacotherapies in the 1990s, the natural history of PAH was extremely poor. Median survival in adults was 2.8 years with 1-, 3-, and 5-year survival rates of 68%, 48%, and 34% [24]. Pediatric outcomes were even worse with a median survival of only 10 months [25]. In the modern therapeutic era, survival rates have improved although PAH continues to be associated with high morbidity and mortality. Adults with newly diagnosed PAH who were included in the REVEAL registry had 1-, 3-, and 5- year respective survivals of 90.4%, 76.2%, and 65.4% [24]. Pediatric survival was found to have similarly improved to 96%, 84%, and 74%, at 1, 3, and 5 years [23].

Populations at Risk of Developing PH

PH is seen in association with numerous disease processes, and this increased risk of developing PH must always be kept in mind. Several barriers exist in effectively diagnosing PH in these patient groups. The presenting symptoms of PH are often nonspecific and depend on the age of the patients. Infants may present with feeding difficulties, tachypnea, poor growth, and a failure to meet developmental milestones. Common symptoms in older children include exertional dyspnea and fatigue, chest pain, lightheadedness, and syncope [25]. Patients may delay seeking treatment, and symptoms are commonly misdiagnosed at initial presentation. In the REVEAL study, the average time from the onset of symptoms to diagnosis was 33 months [26]. Additionally, many patients will be under the care of clinicians who do not routinely treat PH (e.g., patients with sickle cell disease who are primarily cared for by hematologists), and there are limited disease-specific screening guidelines for these patient groups.

Heritable PAH

Several genes have been associated with the development of PAH, the most significant of which is the bone morphogenic protein receptor II gene (BMPR2). Heterozygous mutations of BMPR2 are associated with 80% of cases of familial PAH and are found in 10–20% of sporadic (presumed idiopathic) cases [27]. Most BMPR2 mutations are inherited in an autosomal dominant manner, but disease penetrance is low. Patients with BMPR2 mutations carry a lifetime risk of PAH of 10–20%, and there can be significant differences in penetrance even within members of the same family [8, 28]. For patients who go on to develop PAH, the presence of the BMPR2 mutation has prognostic implications and is associated with an increased risk of death or need for lung transplantation. Current guidelines recommend screening patients with IPAH and first-degree family members of patients with known heritable PAH mutations. Given the potential psychosocial impact of a positive test, genetic counseling before and after testing is paramount [8]. Patients may also be concerned about insurance and employment implications. In the United States, the Genetic Information Nondiscrimination Act (GINA) was passed in 2008 and protects patients against insurance and employment discrimination based on genetic information [29]. There is general agreement that asymptomatic carriers of the disease should undergo periodic screening for PAH, although the optimal screening frequency in this population remains unclear [8, 28].

Congenital Heart Disease

All patients with CHD and systemic to pulmonary (left to right) shunts are at risk of developing PH. In the REVEAL study, 36% of children and 10% of adults had underlying CHD [22, 23]. The risk and timing of the development of PAH depend on both the size and location of the intracardiac shunt. Lesions that are distal to the tricuspid valve (e.g., ventricular septal defects, atrioventricular septal defects, truncus arteriosus) expose the pulmonary vascular bed to excess flow and pressure, and irreversible pulmonary vascular changes can be seen beginning in early infancy. Conversely, pre-tricuspid valve shunts (e.g., atrial septal defects) expose the pulmonary arteries only to excess flow, and the development of PAH may not be seen until the fifth or sixth decade of life [30]. In addition, patients who have undergone repair or palliation may still be at risk for development of PAH later in life, particularly patients who have undergone single ventricle palliation.

Unfortunately, the majority of young adults with CHD fail to transition appropriately, and lapses in care are common. A multicenter survey of adult CHD (ACHD) patients revealed that, beginning at an average age of 20 years, 42% experienced a lapse in care of greater than 3 years and 8% experienced a lapse greater than 10 years [31]. The reasons for this are multifactorial. Most often, patients become lost to follow-up either because they are feeling well or because they did not know continued follow-up was required [31]. There is also a significant shortage of ACHD-trained cardiologists to care for the rapidly growing ACHD population, which now outnumber pediatric CHD patients by more than 2:1 [32]. Ongoing efforts to improve transition and continuous care for patients with CHD include expanded patient education programs, formalized training for cardiologists who wish to specialize in ACHD, and an accreditation process to designate expert ACHD programs as Comprehensive Care Centers.

Sickle Cell Disease

PH occurs in about 10% of patients with sickle cell disease (SCD) [33, 34]. The pathophysiology of PH in SCD patients is multifactorial and remains incompletely understood. Numerous mechanisms have been proposed, with general agreement that chronic intravascular hemolysis, hypoxia-induced lung injury, and thromboembolic disease all play significant roles [35, 36]. Histopathologic lung samples from patients with SCD patients show features of PAH, chronic thromboembolic PH (CTEPH), and pulmonary veno-occlusive disease (PVOD) [35]. On heart catheterization, patients typically have an elevated cardiac output in the setting of their chronic anemia, with only mild elevations in pulmonary pressures and PVR. Given this profile, it has been proposed that a PVR of ≥ 2 Wu be considered abnormal in SCD patients [37, 38]. The presence of PH in SCD is associated with significantly increased mortality, upward of 5–10 times that of patients without PH [38].

Echocardiogram is the most frequently employed screening tool for PH. The peak velocity of the tricuspid regurgitation (TR) jet, a surrogate for systolic pulmonary artery pressure, is elevated in about 30–40% of SCD patients [33, 39]. A TRJ ≥ 2.5 m/sec is considered abnormally elevated, although only a minority of patients with a TR jet of 2.5–2.9 m/sec will have PH on cardiac catheterization [35]. This number is increased in patients who have other markers of PH; the positive predictive value of an elevated TR jet increases from 25% to 62% in the setting of an elevated NT-proBNP (> 164.5 pg/mL) or reduced 6-minute walk distance (< 333 m) [35, 40]. More than 50% of SCD patients with a TRJ > 2.9 m/sec, regardless of symptoms, will have PH [35, 39].

Routine screening for PH in patients with SCD is essential. The basis of this screening should be a careful history and physical exam for signs and symptoms of PH. Routine echocardiogram screening every 1–3 years may be considered and is supported by the American Thoracic Society [38]. However, there is a lack of robust data supporting this, and the American Society of Hematology favors echocardiogram screening primarily in patients with signs or symptoms of PH and patients with associated comorbidities or disease complications known to be associated with PH (e.g., connective tissue disease) [39].

Human Immunodeficiency Virus

There are approximately 1 million people living in the United States (US) with human immunodeficiency virus (HIV). Pediatric patients make up a minority of this population (< 1%), with a significant increase in prevalence seen in the young adult population [41]. Global HIV statistics are starkly different. Nearly 40 million people, 1.7 million of which are children, are living with HIV. The majority of these patients live in developing countries [42]. While the prevalence of PAH in patients with HIV is overall low at about 0.5%, this represents a risk several hundreds of times above that of the general population [43–45]. The underlying mechanisms by which HIV leads to PAH are poorly understood, but histologically the features are the same as in patients with idiopathic PAH [43]. No guidelines exist for screening patients with HIV for PAH, but the development of symptoms should prompt early referral and further evaluation.

Bronchopulmonary Dysplasia

The incidence of PH in premature infants (born at ≤ 28 weeks) with bronchopulmonary dysplasia (BPD) is about 40%; it is the most common cause of pediatric PH due to lung disease [46, 47]. Pulmonary vein stenosis is seen with increased frequency in BPD patients and may further compound the risk of developing PH [48]. PH in infants with BPD is associated with high mortality. In the majority of patients who survive, PH typically resolves over time. However, evidence of persistent pulmonary vascular abnormalities have been seen in long-term follow-up, and PH may reoccur in early adulthood [48, 49]. Additionally, older children and teens with a history of prematurity and BPD have persistent reductions in lung function and increased respiratory morbidities [50]. Data on adult BPD survivors are limited but have shown that these changes also persist into adulthood [51, 52]. Specifically, adults have been shown to have reduced lung function and impaired quality of life.

Considerations for Young Adults with PAH

The Need for Transition

In 1984, US Surgeon General C. Everett Koop, MD, hosted an invitational conference entitled, "Youth with Disability: The Transition Years" [53, 54]. This marked the first major acknowledgment that the healthcare system did not appropriately care for aging young adults with special healthcare needs. In a subsequent position paper, the Society for Adolescent Medicine defined transition as "the purposeful, planned movement of adolescents and young adults with chronic physical and medical conditions from child-centered to adult-oriented health-care systems [54]." Central to this process is the evolution of the patient from a passive to active participant in his or her medical management, ultimately taking on the symbolic role of *CEO* of his or her own healthcare [55, 56]. There is substantial evidence that PAH patients who are well-informed, engaged, and involved in the medical decision-making process have better healthcare outcomes [57–59]. Thus, taking ownership of one's healthcare is critical to the successful management of PAH patients.

Transition Timing

The American Academy of Pediatrics, American Academy of Family Physicians, and American College of Physicians endorse the beginning of the transition process between the ages of 12 and 14 years, with a goal of transfer of care to an adult provider in the 18–21 year age range [55]. The Pulmonary Hypertension Association (PHA), a major international patient advocacy group (www.phassociation.org), supports this transition timing for patients with PH. Institutions caring for PAH patients should have a standard transition protocol in place. It is important that there be inherent flexibility in these protocols, so that they may be adapted to a patient's developmental status [60–62]. Patients must demonstrate appropriate physical and emotional maturity for successful transfer into the adult care environment [31].

Patient Engagement and Quality of Life

In 2014, the US Food and Drug Administration (FDA) described PAH as a disease that, "can rapidly take a significant physical and emotional told on a patient's qualify of life, routine, and the ability of patients to engage in the activities of daily

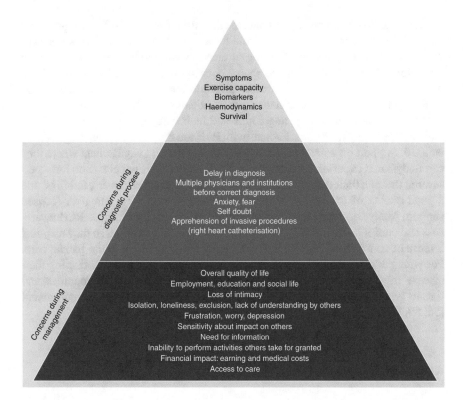

Fig. 10.2 "Tip of the iceberg" model of clinician versus patient that used indicators of health and quality of life. (Reproduced with permission of the © ERS 2020: McGoon et al. [59]. Published 24 January 2019)

living" [63]. This was the conclusion after conducting a public meeting with PAH patients to gain their insight on the disease process. Understanding patient insight is a necessity, and there is often a disconnection between what the provider and patient see as important components of quality of life. Clinicians typically judge disease severity based on objective measures such as symptomatology, biomarkers, and echocardiogram assessment. McGoon and colleagues have described these parameters as the "tip of the iceberg" when one considers the underlying physical, emotional, and psychosocial effects faced by patients and their caregivers (Fig. 10.2) [59]. It is important that both the patient and provider communicate their goals and concerns with one another and each understands the other's perspective.

As part of the transition process, patients are taken from a passive role to an active participant in their own healthcare. When surveyed, the majority of PAH patients express a desire for further information and a more engaged role in their medical care [64]. Patients who participate in a process of shared decision-making with their medical team demonstrate better healthcare outcomes and improved satisfaction [57]. They are more likely to seek out information, make positive lifestyle changes, voice concerns about their medical care, and demonstrate better coping skills [57, 58]. The burden is on the provider to determine how information is best received and how to encourage patients to take on a more active role. Few providers have formal training in this involved and time-consuming process. Transition programs may wish to consider providing further education to their team members on improving patient engagement and shared decision-making [57, 59]. A multidisciplinary team that includes a dedicated transition nurse, social work support, and mental health services can also help support patients through this process.

It is also important that young adults and their caregivers be referred early to patient support organizations. Patients with PAH are frequently left feeling socially isolated. Support organizations are a key source of patient engagement where they can find shared experiences and be inspired by other PAH patients who have persevered through their disease and gone on to have successful careers, families, and a good quality of life. Many of these organizations also offer caregiver-focused support. Many involved patients also participate in activities to raise PAH awareness and contribute to registry studies and research trials; in doing so they may feel a sense of contributing back to the community and improving future patient care. For young adults who feel uncomfortable attending meetings and discussing their disease in person, these associations offer numerous online communities and forums where patients can engage others within a more comfortable environment [58, 59, 65].

Access to Expert Care

The introduction of intravenous epoprostenol in 1995 marked the beginning of a new era of treatment for patients with PAH. At that time, the use of advanced PAH therapies was delegated to a handful of experienced medical centers with expertise in PAH treatment. In the decade that followed, treatment options expanded, and the first oral agents became available (bosentan and sildenafil). As awareness of the disease grew and medication options became more widely available, the treatment paradigm shifted away from these expert centers, toward individual providers who often had little to no experience treating PAH [66–68]. Predictably, this has been a detriment to the care of PH patients, many of whom are subject to incomplete evaluations and inappropriate use of medications. Worse survival outcomes have been seen in patients with PAH cared for outside of expert centers; they are frequently maintained on oral agents despite their clinical status warranting the initiation of intravenous prostacyclin therapy [69]. The multicenter RePHerral study evaluated the accuracy of PH diagnoses and use of PAH pharmacotherapies in patients being referred to tertiary PH centers. Out of a total of 140 patients, 32/98 (32%) patients who had already received diagnoses of PH or PAH were found to be misdiagnosed. Additionally, 59% of patients referred had not previously undergone hemodynamic catheterization, which after being performed led to alternative diagnoses in 89% of these patients. Perhaps most staggering of all, 30% of referred patients had already been prescribed PAH pharmacotherapies, and more than half of patients were receiving therapies that conflicted with published guidelines [66, 70]. In the

Wijeratne study, oral PAH agents were frequently prescribed to patients with Group 2 and Group 3 disease [15]. The inappropriate use of PAH pharmacotherapies presents a serious risk of harm to patient and substantially increases unnecessary healthcare expenditures. The issue was brought into the national spotlight in 2014 when it was chosen as one of the top 5 pulmonary issues as part of the American Board of Internal Medicine's "Choosing Wisely" campaign [71].

These concerns were also recognized by the Scientific Leadership Council of the PHA. In 2011, they conceptualized an accreditation process for designating PH Care Centers (PHCCs) in the US. PHCC accreditation recognizes those expert centers that have the appropriate knowledge and infrastructure to deliver standardized care and guideline-based treatment to patients with PH. The PHA had multiple objectives in mind in creating this accreditation process, including raising disease awareness, increasing access to appropriate care, and fostering research and quality-improvement collaboratives, among centers [26, 66]. However, their primary goal was to improve the quality of care given to patients with PH and, ultimately, to improve patient outcomes [26]. The PHA recognizes two levels of PHCCs, Centers of Comprehensive Care (CCCs) and Regional Clinical Programs (RCPs), the latter of which has to meet less rigorous criteria and represents a program equipped to diagnose and initiate treatment in most patients who do not require parenteral therapies. A comprehensive list of program requirements can be found on the PHA website, referenced above. As of March 2020, there were 59 adult CCCs, 13 adult RCPs, and 8 pediatric CCCs [72].

As there are only a handful of pediatric PHCCs, the majority of pediatric PH patients receive care at non-accredited centers. Often, they are centers with one or a small group of providers with sufficient expertise in treating pediatric PH. Pediatric PH patients face additional challenges compared to adults with PH. The evidence base in children is very limited, and the majority of data regarding the evaluation and care of pediatric PH are extrapolated from adult management. Over the past several years, the United States and Europe have each released pediatric PH guidelines, representing a significant step forward in the standardization of care for children with PH [8, 73]. As part of the transition process, an appropriate adult PH provider should be identified early. This is especially important for young adults who will be relocating for school or work to a new environment. An adult provider at a PHCC is ideal but often not practical due to distance, in which case a local adult provider should have an established relationship with a PHCC to refer patients with advanced disease as needed. Insurance may also play a role in dictating which providers a patient can see. Some patients may receive routine care from both their local provider whom they see regularly and by a PHCC provider whom they see infrequently as needed. With the increasing use of telemedicine, it is also possible for patients to have all required testing done locally and undergo remote expert consultation and follow-up. Prior to the transfer of care, complete medical records should be sent to the adult provider, in addition to which the pediatric and adult providers should meet to discuss the patient. The pediatric provider should also follow up after the patient's first visit with their adult provider to ensure successful transfer [74].

The Burden of PAH Treatment

The treatment of PAH has evolved substantially over the past 30 years, prior to which no PAH-specific therapies were available to patients. There are now five classes of PAH pharmacotherapeutic agents and a total of 14 medications approved by the FDA for adult PAH treatment (Table 10.2). Of note, with the exception of bosentan, none are FDA-approved for pediatric use. Bosentan received FDA

Table 10.2 Targeted PAH medications, dosing, and common side effects

Medication class	Medication	Route	Dose/titration	Adverse effects
Phosphodiesterase-5 inhibitors	Sildenafil (Revatio)	Oral	20 mg TID	Headache, flushing, nasal congestion, dizziness, hypotension, peripheral edema, dyspepsia, diarrhea, myalgia, back pain, sensorineural hearing loss, ischemic optic neuropathy, priapism Co-administration with nitrates is contraindicated
	Tadalafil (Adcirca)	Oral	40 mg QD	Similar to sildenafil Co-administration with nitrates is contraindicated
Endothelin receptor antagonists	Bosentan (Tracleer)	Oral	Initial 62.5 mg BID Maintenance 125 mg BID	Abdominal pain, vomiting, fatigue, headache, edema, flushing, nasal congestion, anemia, decreased sperm count Risk of dose-related increases in liver enzymes Contraindicated in hepatic impairment (monitoring required) Caution with concomitant CYP3A4 inducers and inhibitors Teratogenic
	Ambrisentan (Letairis)	Oral	Initial 5 mg QD Maintenance 10 mg QD	Similar to bosentan Lower risk of liver enzyme elevation Teratogenic
	Macitentan (Opsumit)	Oral	10 mg QD	Similar to bosentan Lower risk of liver enzyme elevation Teratogenic

Table 10.2 (continued)

Medication class	Medication	Route	Dose/titration	Adverse effects
Prostacyclins	Epoprostenol [90] (Flolan, Veletri)	IV	Initial, 2 ng/kg/min Increase by 2 ng/kg/min in increments of at least 15 minutes Maintenance, determined by tolerability	Nausea, flushing, headache, diarrhea, rash, jaw discomfort, thrombocytopenia Hypotension and bleeding with concomitant use of anticoagulants, platelet inhibitors, or vasodilators
	Iloprost (Ventavis)	Inhaled	Initial, 2.5 μg 6 times per day Maintenance, 5 μg 9 times per day	Cough, wheeze, flushing, headache, jaw pain, diarrhea, rash, hypotension May exacerbate reactive airways disease
	Treprostinil [91] (Remodulin, Tyvaso, Orenitram)	IV/subcutaneous	Initial, 1.25 ng/kg/min Maintenance, determined by tolerability	Flushing, headache, nausea, diarrhea, musculoskeletal pain, rash, hypotension, thrombocytopenia, hypokalemia, pain at injection site
		Oral	Initial, 0.25 mg BID or 0.125 mg TID Increase by 0.25 mg or 0.5 mg BID or 0.125 mg TID, not more than every 3–4 days Maintenance, determined by tolerability	Hypotension and bleeding with concomitant use of anticoagulants, platelet inhibitors, or vasodilators
		Inhaled	Initial, 18 μg QID	May exacerbate reactive airway disease at higher doses
Soluble guanylate cyclase stimulator	Riociguat (Adempas)	Oral	Initial, 0.5–1 mg T ID Maintenance, 2.5 mg TID	Headache, dizziness, dyspepsia, nausea, diarrhea, anemia, hypotension, vomiting, gastrointestinal reflux, constipation Co-administration with nitrates and/or PDE-5 inhibitors is contraindicated Teratogenic

(continued)

Table 10.2 (continued)

Medication class	Medication	Route	Dose/titration	Adverse effects
Prostacyclin receptor agonist	Selexipag [92] (Uptravi)	Oral	Initial, 200 mcg BID Maintenance, 1600 mcg BID or highest dose tolerated	Headache, diarrhea, jaw pain, nausea, myalgia, vomiting, extremity pain, flushing, arthralgia, anemia, rash, decreased appetite Contraindicated with concurrent use of CYP2C8 inhibitors

Adapted by permission from: Springer Nature. Ezekian and Hill [94]

approval in 2017 for children 3 years of age and older. The remaining therapies, in particular sildenafil, are frequently used off-label in the pediatric population, with safety and efficacy extrapolated from adult studies [75].

PAH pharmacotherapies are complex, and multiple patient-specific considerations need to be taken into account by prescribers. All PAH medications require prior authorization, and the availability of certain therapies may be limited by a patient's insurance company. Even when therapies are approved and covered, many patients are left with prohibitively high costs. Without insurance, the average whole-sale cost of generic oral sildenafil, the least expensive prescription PAH therapy, is $563 per month. Parenteral prostanoids can cost as much as $14,000 per month [76]. On average, PAH patients pay $2000 a year in out-of-pocket pharmacy costs [77]. Patients and parents should be aware of these costs and coverage issues when making decisions about changes to insurance coverage. Under the Affordable Care Act, young adults may remain on their parents' insurance until age 26. Patients who will be losing their coverage, such as those aging out of government insurance programs, will need to plan in advance to avoid gaps in coverage. Many pharmaceutical companies offer patient assistance programs that provide additional cost coverage for patients over the age of 18. As part of the transition process, patients should be able to demonstrate knowledge of who their insurance provider is, where they get their medications and supplies from, and how to order their medications.

These medications can lead to substantial improvements in patients' PAH-related symptoms and functional class, but their use also comes with significant trade-offs. Side effects are common and can be significant, and medication use may be complex and time-consuming. Common side effects include flushing, headaches, nose bleeds, dizziness, nausea, diarrhea, and bone pain. Thus, between the disease and the medications, patients are seldom symptom-free [63]. Many PAH medications require frequent dosing and can be cumbersome for patients to take. Sildenafil and riociguat are dosed three times a day, and nebulized iloprost must be inhaled six to nine times per day. Patients on some endothelial receptor antagonists (ERAs) are required to get monthly liver function tests, and female patients who are of reproductive age must be on birth control and get monthly pregnancy tests [78]. Patients with advanced PAH (WHO functional class III/IV) typically require treatment with intravenous (IV) prostanoids therapies, either epoprostenol or treprostinil. Parenteral administration requires central line placement, and patients must wear an infusion pump that continuously delivers drug. The use of these medications requires substantial time and responsibility on the part of the patient. Patients must be able to reconstitute the medication and fill their pump cassette appropriately. Some formulations can be prepared up to a week ahead of time, while others must be mixed every 24–48 hours. Patients must also be savvy enough to program dose adjustments into their pumps as instructed by their provider. Abrupt cessation of therapy, either due to running out of medication or central line complications, is an emergency and can precipitate a PH crisis. Traveling requires appropriate planning, and the patient must take sufficient spare equipment [79, 80]. Patients are also subject to central catheter complications, including infection and thrombus, and must be shown how to care for their IV line. Patients on established therapy will receive mail-order shipments of their supplies, which allows these patients to live in more remote areas of the country if needed. These patients should be given information and contact numbers that local emergency rooms, who may not be familiar with these PAH medications, can use for assistance [79].

Employment

Patients frequently express fears about what a diagnosis of PAH means for future employment. The majority of PAH patients and their caregivers report that the disease has an impact on their work ability. They are frequently forced to cut back hours, seek accommodations, take sick leave, change careers, and apply for medical disability. A significant loss of household income is frequently experienced [81, 82]. Globally, employment rates for persons with disabilities are significantly lower than in the general population [83]. In other disease states, it has been shown that structured career counseling and employment advice are associated with higher rates of employment [84]. Patients should also be made aware of workplace antidiscrimination laws, which exist in the United States and in many countries throughout the world, to protect persons with disabilities [83, 85]. Young adults with PAH must be educated on activities and career choices that are safe for them to pursue, with an understanding that their medical needs may change over time. For those with more advanced disease and significant exertional limitations, there are many work options available today that are either more sedentary in nature or permit working from home [65].

Intimacy, Pregnancy, and Contraception

Personal relationships and physical intimacy can be a challenge for both PAH patients and their partners. Anxiety, depression, and poor self-image are common in patients with chronic illnesses, including those with PAH [64]. Additionally, partners of patients often cite concerns over their physical ability to be sexually intimate or that sexual intimacy may make them ill [64, 81]. Clinicians should actively address these topics, as patients may feel a sense of embarrassment in bringing these issues up themselves.

One of the most difficult things to address in patients with PAH is pregnancy. Pregnancy is poorly tolerated in women with PH, and they are among the highest-risk group for maternal and fetal complications, including death. Right heart failure is commonly seen, and women starting pregnancy with depressed right ventricular function have a worse prognosis [86]. Antepartum and postpartum mortality rates range from 16% to 30% [87]. Rates as high as 20–50% are seen in women with baseline cyanosis, such as in Eisenmenger patients [86, 87]. The prognosis for the fetus is equally poor with rates of fetal loss as high as 50% [86]. Due to these risks, pregnancy is contraindicated in women with PAH, and when pregnancy occurs, pregnancy termination should be strongly considered [86, 87].

Extensive education and counseling regarding pregnancy risks, avoidance of pregnancy, and appropriate methods of contraception should be provided to patients and their families. Ideally, this should be done at the time of PAH diagnosis, with recognition that reinforcement may be required later in life as patients form relationships and more strongly consider having a family. The PHA has resources to help patients consider and navigate adoption [65]. In prepubescent females, these discussions may be done with the parents alone. As the patient begins puberty, the topic should be introduced in a manner appropriate for the patient's age and maturity level. Certain PAH pharmacotherapies are teratogenic (all endothelin receptor antagonists and riociguat) and require that female patients who can become pregnant be enrolled in the Risk Evaluation and Mitigation Strategy (REMS) program. The REMS program requires a monthly pregnancy test and appropriate contraception use [88]. Additionally, PAH is associated with a prothrombotic state, and methods of contraception that further increase the risk of thrombosis (such as estrogen-containing contraceptives) should be avoided [89].

As part of the family planning process, both men and women with IPAH or a heritable PAH should undergo genetic counseling and consider testing for genetic mutations associated with PAH. As previously discussed, the BMPR2 mutation is the most common associated with heritable PAH but is associated with low disease penetrance. Therefore, the prognostic value of testing must be weighed carefully against the implications of a positive test. Should a child develop clinical disease, there may be self-blame on the part of the parent who passed on the gene, and parents may be predisposed to treat their child as medically fragile in the face of a potential future illness [8].

Conclusions

PAH is a progressive and often unpredictable disease the affects all aspects of a patient's life. An increasing number of patients are being treated outside of expert centers; they often receive suboptimal care and treatment that is contradictory to published guidelines. The complexity of the disease requires a dedicated transition team to provide high-quality education, understand patient concerns, and encourage patient engagement. This is best achieved through a multidisciplinary team and with early engagement by patients and their caregivers in PH support groups.

References

1. Lammers AE, Apitz C, Zartner P, Hager A, Dubowy KO, Hansmann G. Diagnostics, monitoring and outpatient care in children with suspected pulmonary hypertension/paediatric pulmonary hypertensive vascular disease. Expert consensus statement on the diagnosis and treatment of paediatric pulmonary hypertension. The European Paediatric Pulmonary Vascular Disease Network, endorsed by ISHLT and DGPK. Heart. 2016;102 Suppl 2:ii1–13.
2. Kovacs G, Berghold A, Scheidl S, Olschewski H. Pulmonary arterial pressure during rest and exercise in healthy subjects: a systematic review. Eur Respir J. 2009;34(4):888–94.
3. Simonneau G, Montani D, Celermajer DS, Denton CP, Gatzoulis MA, Krowka M, et al. Haemodynamic definitions and updated clinical classification of pulmonary hypertension. Eur Respir J. 2019;53(1):1–13.
4. Assad TR, Maron BA, Robbins IM, Xu M, Huang S, Harrell FE, et al. Prognostic effect and longitudinal hemodynamic assessment of borderline pulmonary hypertension. JAMA Cardiol. 2017;2(12):1361–8.
5. Vos T, Abajobir AA, Abate KH, Abbafati C, Abbas KM, Abd-Allah F, et al. Global, regional, and national incidence, prevalence, and years lived with disability for 328 diseases and injuries for 195 countries, 1990–2016: a systematic analysis for the Global Burden of Disease Study 2016. Lancet. 2017;390(10100):1211–59.
6. Maron BA, Hess E, Maddox TM, Opotowsky AR, Tedford RJ, Lahm T, et al. Association of borderline pulmonary hypertension with mortality and hospitalization in a large patient cohort: insights from the veterans affairs clinical assessment, reporting, and tracking program. Circulation. 2016;133(13):1240–8.
7. Galie N, Humbert M, Vachiery JL, Gibbs S, Lang I, Torbicki A, et al. 2015 ESC/ERS guidelines for the diagnosis and treatment of pulmonary hypertension: the joint task force for the diagnosis and treatment of pulmonary hypertension of the European Society of Cardiology (ESC) and the European Respiratory Society (ERS): endorsed by: Association for European Paediatric and Congenital Cardiology (AEPC), International Society for Heart and Lung Transplantation (ISHLT). Eur Respir J. 2015;46(4):903–75.
8. Abman SH, Hansmann G, Archer SL, Ivy DD, Adatia I, Chung WK, et al. Pediatric pulmonary hypertension: guidelines from the American Heart Association and American Thoracic Society. Circulation. 2015;132(21):2037–99.
9. Cerro MJ, Abman S, Diaz G, Freudenthal AH, Freudenthal F, Harikrishnan S, et al. A consensus approach to the classification of pediatric pulmonary hypertensive vascular disease: report from the PVRI pediatric taskforce, Panama 2011. Pulm Circ. 2011;1(2):286–98.
10. Foshat M, Boroumand N. The evolving classification of pulmonary hypertension. Arch Pathol Lab Med. 2017;141(5):696–703.
11. Ivy DD, Abman SH, Barst RJ, Berger RM, Bonnet D, Fleming TR, et al. Pediatric pulmonary hypertension. J Am Coll Cardiol. 2013;62(25 Suppl):D117–26.
12. Rosenzweig EB, Abman SH, Adatia I, Beghetti M, Bonnet D, Haworth S, et al. Paediatric pulmonary arterial hypertension: updates on definition, classification, diagnostics and management. Eur Respir J. 2019;53(1):1801916.
13. Hoeper MM, Humbert M, Souza R, Idrees M, Kawut SM, Sliwa-Hahnle K, et al. A global view of pulmonary hypertension. Lancet Respir Med. 2016;4(4):306–22.

14. Graham BB, Bandeira AP, Morrell NW, Butrous G, Tuder RM. Schistosomiasis-associated pulmonary hypertension: pulmonary vascular disease: the global perspective. Chest. 2010;137(6 Suppl):20S–9S.
15. Wijeratne DT, Lajkosz K, Brogly SB, Lougheed MD, Jiang L, Housin A, et al. Increasing incidence and prevalence of World Health Organization groups 1 to 4 pulmonary hypertension: a population-based cohort study in Ontario, Canada. Circ Cardiovasc Qual Outcomes. 2018;11:e003973.
16. van Loon RL, Roofthooft MT, Hillege HL, ten Harkel AD, van Osch-Gevers M, Delhaas T, et al. Pediatric pulmonary hypertension in the Netherlands: epidemiology and characterization during the period 1991 to 2005. Circulation. 2011;124(16):1755–64.
17. Ivy D. Pulmonary hypertension in children. Cardiol Clin. 2016;34(3):451–72.
18. Davidson LM, Berkelhamer SK. Bronchopulmonary dysplasia: chronic lung disease of infancy and long-term pulmonary outcomes. J Clin Med. 2017;6(1):4.
19. del Cerro Marin MJ, Sabate Rotes A, Rodriguez Ogando A, Mendoza Soto A, Quero Jimenez M, Gavilan Camacho JL, et al. Assessing pulmonary hypertensive vascular disease in childhood. Data from the Spanish registry. Am J Respir Crit Care Med. 2014;190(12):1421–9.
20. Hansmann G. Pulmonary hypertension in infants, children, and young adults. J Am Coll Cardiol. 2017;69(20):2551–69.
21. McGoon MD, Humbert M. Pulmonary arterial hypertension: epidemiology and registries. Advances in Pulmonary Hypertension. 2014;13:21–6.
22. McGoon MD, Miller DP. REVEAL: a contemporary US pulmonary arterial hypertension registry. Eur Respir Rev. 2012;21(123):8–18.
23. Barst RJ, McGoon MD, Elliott CG, Foreman AJ, Miller DP, Ivy DD. Survival in childhood pulmonary arterial hypertension: insights from the registry to evaluate early and long-term pulmonary arterial hypertension disease management. Circulation. 2012;125(1):113–22.
24. Farber HW, Miller DP, Poms AD, Badesch DB, Frost AE, Muros-Le Rouzic E, et al. Five-year outcomes of patients enrolled in the REVEAL registry. Chest. 2015;148(4):1043–54.
25. Takatsuki S, Ivy DD. Current challenges in pediatric pulmonary hypertension. Semin Respir Crit Care Med. 2013;34(5):627–44.
26. Mathai SC. A rare opportunity in a rare disease. Adv Pulm Hypertens. 2018;16:175–8.
27. Kiely DG, Lawrie A, Humbert M. Screening strategies for pulmonary arterial hypertension. Eur Heart J Suppl. 2019;21(Suppl K):K9–K20.
28. Lau EM, Humbert M, Celermajer DS. Early detection of pulmonary arterial hypertension. Nat Rev Cardiol. 2015;12(3):143–55.
29. Genetic Information Nondiscrimination Act of 2008, Pub L. No. 110-233, 122, Stat. 881.
30. Rosenzweig EB, Barst RJ. Congenital heart disease and pulmonary hypertension: pharmacology and feasibility of late surgery. Prog Cardiovasc Dis. 2012;55(2):128–33.
31. Gurvitz M, Valente AM, Broberg C, Cook S, Stout K, Kay J, et al. Prevalence and predictors of gaps in care among adult congenital heart disease patients: HEART-ACHD (the health, education, and access research trial). J Am Coll Cardiol. 2013;61:2180–4.
32. Zaidi AN, Daniels CJ. The Adolescent and Adult with Cogenital Heart Disease. In: Allen HD, Shaddy RE, Penny DJ, Cetta F, Feltes TF, editors. Moss and Adams' heart disease in infants, children, and adolescents: including the fetus and young adult. 9th ed. Philadelphia: Wolters Kulwer; 2016. p. 1559–99.
33. Fonseca GH, Souza R, Salemi VM, Jardim CV, Gualandro SF. Pulmonary hypertension diagnosed by right heart catheterisation in sickle cell disease. Eur Respir J. 2012;39(1):112–8.
34. Mehari A, Gladwin MT, Tian X, Machado RF, Kato GJ. Mortality in adults with sickle cell disease and pulmonary hypertension. JAMA. 2012;307(12):1254–6.
35. Gordeuk VR, Castro OL, Machado RF. Pathophysiology and treatment of pulmonary hypertension in sickle cell disease. Blood. 2016;127(7):820–8.
36. Machado RF, Gladwin MT. Chronic sickle cell lung disease: new insights into the diagnosis, pathogenesis and treatment of pulmonary hypertension. Br J Haematol. 2005;129(4):449–64.

37. Fonseca G, Souza R. Pulmonary hypertension in sickle cell disease. Curr Opin Pulm Med. 2015;21(5):432–7.
38. Klings ES, Machado RF, Barst RJ, Morris CR, Mubarak KK, Gordeuk VR, et al. An official American Thoracic Society clinical practice guideline: diagnosis, risk stratification, and management of pulmonary hypertension of sickle cell disease. Am J Respir Crit Care Med. 2014;189(6):727–40.
39. Liem RI, Lanzkron S, Coates TD, DeCastro L, Desai AA, Ataga KI, et al. American Society of Hematology 2019 guidelines for sickle cell disease: cardiopulmonary and kidney disease. Blood Adv. 2019;3(23):3867–97.
40. Hayes MM, Vedamurthy A, George G, Dweik R, Klings ES, Machado RF, et al. Pulmonary hypertension in sickle cell disease. Ann Am Thorac Soc. 2014;11(9):1488–9.
41. Centers for Disease Control and Prevention. HIV surveillance report, 2018 (Preliminary); vol. 30. http://www.cdc.gov/hiv/library/reports/hiv-surveillance.html. Published November 2019. Accessed 2 Apr 2020. 2018;30.
42. UNAIDS. Global HIV & AIDS statistics - 2019 fact sheet. https://www.unaids.org/en/resources/fact-sheet. Published December 2019. Accessed 2 Apr 2020.
43. Basyal B, Jarrett H, Barnett CF. Pulmonary hypertension in HIV. Can J Cardiol. 2019;35(3):288–98.
44. Bigna JJ, Sime PS, Koulla-Shiro S. HIV related pulmonary arterial hypertension: epidemiology in Africa, physiopathology, and role of antiretroviral treatment. AIDS Res Ther. 2015;12:36.
45. Correale M, Palmiotti GA, Lo Storto MM, Montrone D, Foschino Barbaro MP, Di Biase M, et al. HIV-associated pulmonary arterial hypertension: from bedside to the future. Eur J Clin Invest. 2015;45(5):515–28.
46. Stoll BJ, Hansen NI, Bell EF, Shankaran S, Laptook AR, Walsh MC, Hale EC, Newman NS, Schibler K, Carlo WA, Kennedy KA, Poindexter BB, Finer NN, Ehrenkranz RA, Duara S, Sánchez PJ, O'Shea TM, Goldberg RN, Van Meurs KP, Faix RG, Phelps DL, Frantz ID 3rd, Watterberg KL, Saha S, Das A, Higgins RD, Eunice Kennedy Shriver National Institute of Child Health and Human Development Neonatal Research Network. Bronchopulmonary dysplasia: definition, pathogenesis, and clinical features. Pediatrics. 2010;126:443–56.
47. Awerbach JD, Mallory GB Jr, Kim S, Cabrera AG. Hospital readmissions in children with pulmonary hypertension: a multi-institutional analysis. J Pediatr. 2018;195:95–101 e4.
48. Varghese N, Rios D. Pulmonary hypertension associated with bronchopulmonary dysplasia: a review. Pediatr Allergy Immunol Pulmonol. 2019;32(4):140–8.
49. Altit G, Dancea A, Renaud C, Perreault T, Lands LC, Sant'Anna G. Pathophysiology, screening and diagnosis of pulmonary hypertension in infants with bronchopulmonary dysplasia - a review of the literature. Paediatr Respir Rev. 2017;23:16–26.
50. Fawke J, Lum S, Kirkby J, Hennessy E, Marlow N, Rowell V, et al. Lung function and respiratory symptoms at 11 years in children born extremely preterm: the EPICure study. Am J Respir Crit Care Med. 2010;182(2):237–45.
51. Caskey S, Gough A, Rowan S, Gillespie S, Clarke J, Riley M, et al. Structural and functional lung impairment in adult survivors of bronchopulmonary dysplasia. Ann Am Thorac Soc. 2016;13(8):1262–70.
52. Gough A, Linden M, Spence D, Patterson CC, Halliday HL, McGarvey LP. Impaired lung function and health status in adult survivors of bronchopulmonary dysplasia. Eur Respir J. 2014;43(3):808–16.
53. Blum R. Introduction. Improving transition for adolescents with special health care needs from pediatric to adult-centered health care. Pediatrics. 2002;110:1301–3.
54. Blum RW, Garell D, Hodgman CH, Jorissen TW, Okinow NA, Orr DP, et al. Transition from child-centered to adult health-care systems for adolescents with chronic conditions: a position paper of the Society for Adolescent Medicine. J Adolesc Health. 1993;14:570–6.
55. White P, Cooley W, Transitions Clinical Report Authoring Group, American Academy of Pediatrics, American Academy of Family Physicians, American College of Physicians.

Supporting the health care transition from adolescence to aduthood in the medical home. Pediatrics. 2018;142:e20182587.

56. Kieckhefer G, Trahms C. Supporting development of children with chronic conditions: from compliance toward shared management. Pediatr Nurs. 2000;26:354–63.

57. Actelion Pharmaceuticals Ltd. A holistic approach to patient care in pulmonary arterial hypertension. 2016. Date last accessed: March 2020. Date last updated: January 2016.

58. Graarup J, Ferrari P, Howard LS. Patient engagement and self-management in pulmonary arterial hypertension. Eur Respir Rev. 2016;25(142):399–407.

59. McGoon MD, Ferrari P, Armstrong I, Denis M, Howard LS, Lowe G, et al. The importance of patient perspectives in pulmonary hypertension. Eur Respir J. 2019;53(1):1801919. https://doi.org/10.1183/13993003.01919-2018.

60. Saidi A, Kovacs AH. Developing a transition program from pediatric- to adult-focused cardiology care: practical considerations. Congenit Heart Dis. 2009;4:204–15.

61. Knauth Meadows A, Bosco V, Tong E, Fernandes S, Saidi A. Transition and transfer from pediatric to adult care of young adults with complex congenital heart disease. Curr Cardiol Rep. 2009;11:291–307.

62. Sable C, Foster E, Uzark K, Bjornsen K, Canobbio MM, Connolly HM, et al. Best practices in managing transition to adulthood for adolescents with congenital heart disease: the transition process and medical and psychosocial issues: a scientific statement from the American Heart Association. Circulation. 2011;123:1454–85.

63. Center for Drug Evaluation and Research, U.S. Food and Drug Administration. The voice of the patient: a series of reports from the U.S. Food and Drug Administration's (FDA's) patient-focused drug development initiative; 2014.

64. Guillevin L, Armstrong I, Aldrighetti R, Howard LS, Ryftenius H, Fischer A, et al. Understanding the impact of pulmonary arterial hypertension on patients' and carers' lives. Eur Respir Rev. 2013;22(130):535–42.

65. Actelion Pharmaceuticals. Supporting young adult living with pulmonary arterial hypertension (PAH) in the best practice management of their disease; 2017.

66. Chakinala M, McGoon M. Pulmonary hypertension care centers. Advances in Pulmonary Hypertension. 2014;12:175–8.

67. Talwar A, Garcia JGN, Tsai H, Moreno M, Lahm T, Zamanian RT, et al. Health disparities in patients with pulmonary arterial hypertension: a blueprint for action. An official American Thoracic Society statement. Am J Respir Crit Care Med. 2017;196(8):e32–47.

68. Oudiz RJ. Evolution in PH care: 3 decades of milestones. Advances in Pulmonary Hypertension. 2018;16:165–9.

69. Badagliacca R, Pezzuto B, Poscia R, Mancone M, Papa S, Marcon S, et al. Prognostic factors in severe pulmonary hypertension patients who need parenteral prostanoid therapy: the impact of late referral. J Heart Lung Transplant. 2012;31(4):364–72.

70. Deano RC, Glassner-Kolmin C, Rubenfire M, Frost A, Visovatti S, McLaughlin VV, et al. Referral of patients with pulmonary hypertension diagnoses to tertiary pulmonary hypertension centers: the multicenter RePHerral study. JAMA Intern Med. 2013;173(10):887–93.

71. Wiener RS, Ouellette DR, Diamond E, Fan VS, Maurer JR, Mularski RA, et al. An official American Thoracic Society/American College of Chest Physicians policy statement: the Choosing Wisely top five list in adult pulmonary medicine. Chest. 2014;145(6):1383–91.

72. Pulmonary Hypertension Association. PH Care Centers 2020 [cited Mar 30, 2020]. Available from: https://phassociation.org/phcarecenters/.

73. Hansmann G, Koestenberger M, Alastalo TP, Apitz C, Austin ED, Bonnet D, et al. 2019 updated consensus statement on the diagnosis and treatment of pediatric pulmonary hypertension: the European Pediatric Pulmonary Vascular Disease Network (EPPVDN), endorsed by AEPC, ESPR and ISHLT. J Heart Lung Transplant. 2019;38(9):879–901.

74. Coleman BA, Calderbank M. Transitioning the pediatric pulmonary hypertension patient (advances in pulmonary hypertension). Adv Pulm Hypertens. 2012;11:162–4.

75. Awerbach JD, Krasuski RA, Hill KD. Characteristics of pediatric pulmonary hypertension trials registered on ClinicalTrials.gov. Pulm Circ. 2017;7(2):348–360.
76. Macitentan (Opsumit): for long-term treatment of pulmonary arterial hypertension [Internet]. Ottawa (ON): Canadian Agency for Drugs and Technologies in Health; 2015 Jul. Table 1, Cost comparison table for drugs used for the treatment of pulmonary arterial hypertension. Available from: https://www.ncbi.nlm.nih.gov/books/NBK349251/table/T30/.
77. Sikirica M, Iorga SR, Bancroft T, Potash J. The economic burden of pulmonary arterial hypertension (PAH) in the US on payers and patients. BMC Health Serv Res. 2014;14:676.
78. Grady RM, Eghtesady P. Potts shunt and pediatric pulmonary hypertension: what we have learned. Ann Thorac Surg. 2016;101(4):1539–43.
79. Farber HW, Gin-Sing W. Practical considerations for therapies targeting the prostacyclin pathway. Eur Respir Rev. 2016;25(142):418–30.
80. LeVarge BL, Pomerantsev E, Channick RN. Reliance on end-expiratory wedge pressure leads to misclassification of pulmonary hypertension. Eur Respir J. 2014;44(2):425–34.
81. Zhai Z, Zhou X, Zhang S, Xie W, Wan J, Kuang T, et al. The impact and financial burden of pulmonary arterial hypertension on patients and caregivers: results from a national survey. Medicine (Baltimore). 2017;96(39):e6783.
82. Armstrong I, Billings C, Kiely DG, Yorke J, Harries C, Clayton S, et al. The patient experience of pulmonary hypertension: a large cross-sectional study of UK patients. BMC Pulm Med. 2019;19(1):67.
83. World Health Organization, World Bank. World report on disability; 2011.
84. Crossland DS, Jackson SP, Lyall R, Burn J, O'Sullivan JJ. Employment and advice regarding careers for adults with congenital heart disease. Cardiol Young. 2005;15:391–5.
85. Americans with Disabilities Act of 1990, as amended, Pub. L. No. 110-336 Stat. 12101 (2009).
86. Canobbio MM, Warnes CA, Aboulhosn J, Connolly HM, Khanna A, Koos BJ, et al. Management of pregnancy in patients with complex congenital heart disease: a scientific statement for healthcare professionals from the American Heart Association. Circulation. 2017;135:e50–87.
87. Regitz-Zagrosek V, Roos-Hesselink JW, Bauersachs J, Blomström-Lundqvist C, Cífková R, De Bonis M, et al. 2018 ESC guidelines for the management of cardiovascular diseases during pregnancy. Eur Heart J. 2018;39(34):3165–241.
88. Ambrisentan REMS. Ambrisentan REMS guide for female patients; 2019.
89. Olsson KM, Channick R. Pregnancy in pulmonary arterial hypertension. Eur Respir Rev. 2016;25(142):431–7.
90. Veletri (epoprostenol). Dec 2012. Highlights of prescribing information. https://www.accessdata.fda.gov/drugsatfda_docs/label/2012/022260s005lbl.pdf. Last accessed: April 2020.
91. Orenitram (Treprostinil). Jan 2017. Highlights of prescribing information. https://www.accessdata.fda.gov/drugsatfda_docs/label/2017/203496s006lbl.pdf. Last accessed: April 2020.
92. UPTRAVI (selexipag). Dec 2015. Highlights of prescribing information. https://www.accessdata.fda.gov/drugsatfda_docs/label/2015/207947s000lbl.pdf. Date last accessed: April 2020.
93. Simonneau G, et al. Haemodynamic definitions and updated clinical classification of pulmonary hypertension. Eur Respir J. 2019;53(1):1801913. https://doi.org/10.1183/1399300 3.01913-2018.
94. Ezekian JE, Hill KD. Management of pulmonary arterial hypertension in the pediatric patient. Curr Cardiol Rep. 2019;21(12):162.

Index

© Springer Nature Switzerland AG 2021
C. D. Brown, E. Crowley (eds.), *Transitioning Care from Pediatric to Adult
Pulmonology*, Respiratory Medicine,
https://doi.org/10.1007/978-3-030-68688-8

Printed in the United States
by Baker & Taylor Publisher Services